MEDICARE AND MEDIGAPS

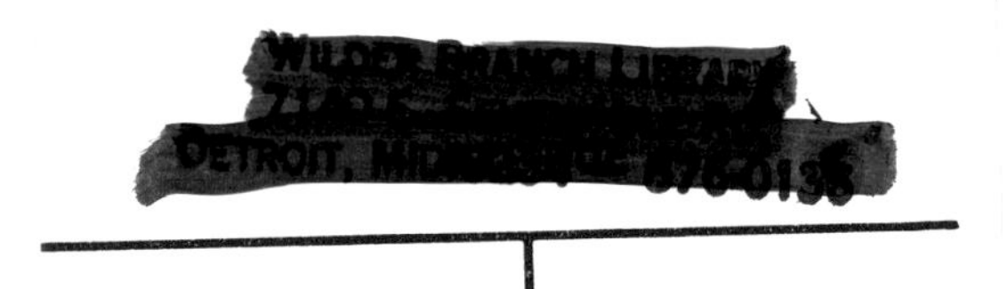

MEDICARE AND MEDIGAPS

A Guide to Retirement Health Insurance

SUSAN HELLMAN
LEONARD H. HELLMAN

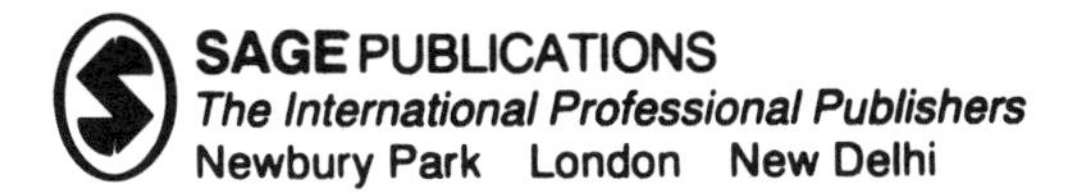
SAGE PUBLICATIONS
The International Professional Publishers
Newbury Park London New Delhi

For information address:

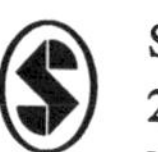

SAGE Publications, Inc.
2455 Teller Road
Newbury Park, California 91320

SAGE Publications Ltd.
6 Bonhill Street
London EC2A 4PU
United Kingdom

SAGE Publications India Pvt. Ltd.
M-32 Market
Greater Kailash I
New Delhi 110 048 India

Printed in the United States of America

Library of Congress Cataloging-in-Publication Data

Hellman, Susan.
Medicare and medigaps : a guide to retirement health insurance / Susan Hellman, Leonard H. Helman.
p. cm.
Includes bibliographical references and index.
ISBN 0-8039-4366-0 (p)
1. Medicare. 2. medigap. I. Hellman, Leonard H. II. Title.
HD7102.U4H435 1991
368.3'2'00296—dc20 91-22012

FIRST PRINTING, 1991

Sage Production Editor: Diane S. Foster

CONTENTS

TABLES

FIGURES

ACKNOWLEDGMENTS

We would like to thank the following people for their invaluable assistance in preparing this book. Without their expertise and their patient willingness to answer questions, it would have been impossible to keep up with the abundance of changing rules and regulations. Many thanks to Mary Lou Amoroso at the Social Security Administration; Frank Szeflinksi and Steve Blake at the Region VIII office of the Health Care Financing Administration; Cindy Hoskins, Jan Popovitch, and Kris Kortekaas of Medicare at Blue Cross/Blue Shield of Colorado; Judie Lenhart of the Colorado Foundation for Medical Care (PRO); the Colorado Division of Insurance; Ezra Yoder of Yoder Eby, Inc.; Jean Bress of Aging and Adult Services at the Colorado Department of Social Services; Greg Fuller of Kaiser Permanente; Richard Ceresko of the Colorado Division of Veterans Affairs; Virginia Mullen of Saint Joseph Hospital; and all the devoted Senior Health Insurance Counseling Program volunteers. A very special thanks to the Comprecare Foundation that faithfully supports health care education.

PREFACE

The subject of Medicare and other health insurance options for older Americans is complicated. Regulations change frequently, making it virtually impossible for consumers to keep up-to-date. Yet 97% of Americans must deal with Medicare when they turn 65. Many people have problems understanding what Medicare does and does not cover and how to select Medicare supplemental insurance. Many are worried about how to protect themselves from the catastrophic costs of long-term care. And many sleepless nights are spent worrying about the overwhelming amounts of paperwork that result from medical claims. Getting assistance from people who know the ropes is not easy.

This book attempts to present in easy-to-understand language an overview of some of the major issues of retirement health insurance. It explains what is covered by Medicare Parts A and B, how to buy insurance that supplements Medicare, and how to deal with the paperwork. We hope this book is useful to those who work with older adults and, perhaps, even to those older adults interested in learning more about the Medicare system. Perhaps one day a book of this type will not be needed. We hope that eventually the health care system in this country will not only be greatly simplified, but that it will be accessible to *all* Americans.

1

MEDICARE

History, Financing, and Eligibility

HISTORY OF MEDICARE PROGRAM

What Is Social Security?

The Social Security Act, passed by Congress in 1935 during President Franklin Roosevelt's first term, along with later related laws, provides for the material needs of individuals and families. Medicare, enacted in 1965, protects aged and disabled persons against the expenses of illnesses that could otherwise exhaust their savings. The Social Security programs are intended to "keep families together, and give children the opportunity to grow up in good health and security." Programs include retirement, survivors, and disability insurance; Medicare; black lung benefits; supplemental security income; unemployment insurance; and public assistance and welfare services such as aid to needy families with children, medical assistance (Medicaid), maternal and child health services, child support enforcement, family and child welfare services, food stamps, and energy assistance. Some of these programs are operated solely by the federal government, and some are operated in cooperation with the individual states.

Note: In 1991 persons between the ages of 65–69 can earn up to $9,720 per year without penalty. For income over that amount, the Social Security cash benefit is reduced by $1 for every $3 earned. Up to age 64, benefits are reduced $1 for every $2 earned over $7,080. Over age 70, there are no Social Security penalties on earned income.

What Is Medicare?

Ninety-seven percent of Americans over 65 have health insurance protection through Medicare. Medicare was enacted by the federal government in 1965, under President Lyndon B. Johnson, as Title XVIII (18) of the Social Security Act. It became effective July 1, 1966. The program entitles persons 65 and over (and their spouses if at least age 65) who have paid into the Social Security system or Railroad Retirement benefits to federal health insurance coverage. It also covers two categories of persons under age 65: those with end-stage renal (kidney) disease and disabled persons who have been receiving Social Security disability benefits for 24 months. Medicare is an entitlement program and is not needs-based like

Medicaid, which is a federal–state program of medical assistance based on need.

Who Administers Medicare?

The Medicare program is delegated to the Department of Health and Human Services (DHHS), which is a department in the executive branch of the federal government. Within DHHS, the Social Security Administration (SSA) is responsible for Medicare eligibility and enrollment, and the Health Care Financing Administration (HCFA) establishes all the rules, regulations, and health-related policies governing the Medicare and Medicaid program. Dr. Louis Sullivan is presently the Secretary of Health and Human Services. Gwendolyn S. King is the Commissioner of the Social Security Administration. Dr. Gail Wilensky is the Health Care Financing Administration Chief.

The HCFA contracts with private insurance companies throughout the country to process Medicare claims. Each state has an *intermediary* (private insurance company that processes Part A claims) and a *carrier* (private insurance company that processes Part B claims).

Social Security personnel will answer questions about enrollment and eligibility. The HCFA a beneficiary services branch or your local Part B Medicare carrier will answer questions about Medicare coverage. If your state has a senior health insurance counseling program, this is also a good resource for Medicare information.

What Kind of Health Care Insurance Does Medicare Provide?

Medicare is divided into two parts: Part A, hospital insurance (HI); and Part B, medical insurance (also called SMI or supplemental medical insurance). Medicare pays a portion, *not all,* of a beneficiary's health care costs. Therefore, many Medicare beneficiaries supplement their coverage with private health insurance or some of the other options discussed in Chapter 4.

When people enroll in Medicare, they do not have to pay a monthly premium for Part A. Part A coverage has been earned through a person's payroll taxes deducted during his or her working years. Part B, however, is voluntary and requires a monthly premium, most often deducted from a person's Social Security check each month. A person can reject Part B and will not have to pay the monthly premium, but this is not advised as will be discussed later in this chapter.

FINANCING MEDICARE

How Is Medicare Funded?

Funds come from payroll taxes, general taxes, interest accumulated from the Health Insurance Trust Funds, and monthly premiums paid by Medicare beneficiaries. In addition, beneficiaries are responsible for paying deductibles and coinsurance amounts.

Where Are the Medicare Funds Kept?

The Health Insurance Trust Funds established under the Social Security Act are comprised of

Federal Hospital Insurance Trust Fund (Part A benefits). A federal hospital insurance trust fund is supported primarily by payroll or earnings tax paid by employers, employees, and self-employed persons. (In 1991 although the maximum annual earnings subject to FICA tax is $53,400, income subject to the Medicare tax is 1.45% on earnings up to $125,000.)

Federal Supplementary Medical Insurance Trust Fund (Part B benefits). A federal supplementary medical insurance trust fund is comprised of enrollees' monthly premiums, general taxes, and trust fund interest. Medicare beneficiaries pay a monthly premium for Part B that increases each year to provide approximately 25% of the funds needed.

Are Unreimbursed Medical Expenses Tax Deductible?

Unreimbursed medical expenses, including private medical insurance premiums and Medicare monthly premiums, can be claimed as itemized deductions if they exceed 7.5% of a person's adjusted gross income.

ELIGIBILITY AND ENROLLMENT

Who Is Eligible for Medicare?

Persons 65 Years Old Who Are Eligible for Social Security Benefits

HUSBAND AND WIFE

Bill is 65 and is filing for Social Security benefits. His wife, Nora, is also eligible for Social Security and retires that same year at age 62. Bill is eligible to enroll in Medicare, but Nora will not be eligible until the first day of the month when she becomes 65.

Elaine, who is 65, never worked outside the home and is not eligible for Social Security benefits on her own record. She is married to Sven who is 60 and who will be eligible for reduced Social Security cash benefits at age 62. Elaine is eligible for Social Security Retirement Benefits and entitled to Medicare based on Sven's record; however, not until he turns 62. (At age 65, Elaine would also be eligible had her younger, eligible spouse become disabled or died prior to age 62.)

WIDOW

Theresa is a widow whose husband died last year at age 63. Theresa will be turning 65 in a few months. She never held a job that paid into social Security. Nevertheless, her late husband was eligible for Social Security benefits. She will be entitled to Medicare at age 65. (If she had contacted the Social Security Administration when her husband died, she could have chosen to receive reduced monthly Social Security cash benefits at that time.)

DIVORCED, REMARRIED

Tony, 68, has been married three times. He was married to his first wife Carla, now 68, for 12 years before they divorced. He was married to Vicki, now 68, for 7 years before they divorced. He thinks his 2-year marriage to Bubbles, now 68, is the real thing. None of the women worked outside the home. Carla and Bubbles are entitled to Medicare under Tony's eligibility, but Vicki is not because she was married to Tony for less than 10 years before divorcing. Bubbles is eligible, even though she has only been married to Tony for 2 years because she is his current wife and has been married to him for over 1 year.

Persons With End-Stage Renal Disease (Can Be Under 65)

Barbara is undergoing kidney dialysis. At age 28, she works and contributes to Social Security through her payroll taxes. She has obtained a certification proving that she requires dialysis. She is eligible for Medicare. If her condition improves so that dialysis is no longer needed, she is entitled to continue Medicare coverage for 12 months after her dialysis is completed.

Persons Under Age 65 Receiving Disability Benefits

Roger, 52, has been unable to work for the past 2 years due to emphysema. He has qualified for Social Security disability income (SSDI). After 24 months on Social Security disability, he will automatically be covered by Medicare. (Disability payments may only be made through age 64, then they convert to Retirement Benefits.)

Some Persons Over Age 65 Who Are Not Eligible for Social Security Can Purchase Medicare

Persons who have not worked long enough to pay into Social Security may be eligible by paying premiums.

Isabelle's mother, Tatiana, who is 65, will be coming to the United States from Holland to live with her daughter. She will become a legal permanent resident of the United States. Because she has not paid into the Social Security system, she is not eligible for any benefits, including Medicare. However, after living here continuously for 5 years, she can purchase Part A (called Premium Hospital Insurance). She is called a "voluntary enrollee" in Part A. She will pay $177 per month in 1991 for Part A and $29.90 per month for Part B. However, she faces a limited 10% penalty that applies only to *voluntary enrollees* who enroll in Part A beyond age 65. There is also a 10% per year continuing penalty for all persons who enroll in Part B beyond age 65 and who are not otherwise exempt. Tatiana can purchase Part B only. If she purchases Part A, she *must* buy Part B.

Persons Over Age 65 Who Qualify Under Special Categories

Hedda was not eligible for Social Security when she turned 65 in 1973. A special "transitional category of automatic eligibility," however, applies to people who turned 65 before 1975 (1974 for women) who had a minimum of three quarters of work credit for work after 1966. Hedda met this requirement and was automatically eligible for Medicare.

Molly turned 65 in 1967. Even though she is not eligible for Social Security, a special rule for those who turned 65 before 1968 makes them automatically eligible for Medicare if they are U.S. citizens or have lawfully lived in the United States for 5 consecutive years prior to applying for Medicare.

How Does a Person Apply for Medicare?

It is best to apply for Medicare any time during the *initial enrollment period,* which includes the 3 months prior to your 65th birth month, the birth month itself, and the 3 months following your 65th birth month combined this is a 7-month period. For those who fail to enroll during the initial enrollment period, there is a *general enrollment period* each year. For those who are still working and continue to be covered by an employer group health plan (either their own or their spouse's), there is a *special enrollment period.* Unless you or your spouse are employed and covered by an employer group health plan, you will find it very hard, if not impossible, to obtain comprehensive health insurance if you do not enroll in Medicare.

Persons Should Apply for Social Security Benefits at Age 65 During the 7 Months Surrounding Their 65th Birthday, Which Is the ***Initial Enrollment Period***

Application during the 3 months preceding a person's 65th birth month. For example, Arvid will be 65 in 3 months and he wants to begin receiving his cash benefits and enroll in Medicare. He may call the national toll-free Social Security line at 1-800-234-5772 to make an appointment to apply or he may go to his local office (he may have to wait unless an appointment has been made). He will be sent a confirmation of this appointment along with information about what documents he will need to bring. He may apply either by telephone or in person at his nearest Social Security office. The documents he may need are his W-2 forms for the past 2 years showing his employer's report of annual earnings as reported to the Internal Revenue Service or, if self-employed, his last two federal income tax returns; his Social Security card; proof of age on a birth certificate, baptismal certificate, or hospital record; or proof of marriage to a spouse who is eligible for benefits if he is not eligible for Social Security.

Coverage will become effective the first day of the month in which Arvid becomes 65. He will automatically be enrolled in Part A *and* Part B unless he voluntarily rejects Part B. Beginning in the month he turns 65, a monthly premium will automatically be taken out of his Social Security check if he elects Part B.

Application during birth month (initial enrollment period). For example, Anna turned 65 several days ago on the first of the month. Realizing she is eligible for benefits, she applies for her Social Security cash benefits and enrolls in Medicare that same month. Her coverage will begin the first day of the month following her 65th birthday.

Application during the 3 months following birth month (still within the initial enrollment period). For example, Harry born in March, was out of the country for the last 6 months and enrolls in Medicare during April, 1 month after he turned 65. His coverage will begin on June 1. If he enrolls in May, his coverage will be effective August 1. If he enrolls in June, which is the last month of his initial enrollment period, coverage will be effective on September 1.

Persons Can Apply for Part A 4 Months or More After Their 65th Birth Month and for Part B During the ***General Enrollment Period***

Application 4 months or more after 65th birth month. For example, Marlon passed his 65th birthday 4 months ago, in August. He can enroll in Part A, which will make him eligible retroactively for the month he was 65. To enroll in Part B, however, he must now wait until the next general enrollment period, which occurs January 1 through March 31 of each year. His part B coverage will begin on July 1. He will pay no penalty for late enrollment since it is within 1 year of his birth month.

Application 1 year or more after 65th birth month. For example, Bert is 67. He did not apply for Medicare 2 years ago when he turned 65, so he enrolls in Part A and his coverage becomes retroactive to the 6th month prior to the month he applied. There is no penalty. Because he now can only apply for Medicare Part B during the first 3 months of a calendar year following his 65th birthday, he does so the following January. Because more than 1 year has elapsed since his 65th birth month, there is a permanent 10% increase added on to his monthly Part B premium.

This 10% penalty is added on for each year a person could have but did not enroll in Part B. It is calculated as a percentage of the enrollment year's

Part B monthly premium and then added on to that year's premium. For example, it might be 20% more than the present monthly premium for a person enrolling 2 years late, or 110% for a person enrolling 11 years late. The maximum penalty in 1991 is 240% or $101.70 per month.

Special enrollment period: This Part B penalty is waived for working persons over 65 who are enrolled in an employer group health plan. The person must, however, enroll in Part B within the 7 months after retiring, or at such time as the employer's health plan ceases.

Persons Already Receiving Social Security Benefits When They Reach 65 Will Automatically Be Enrolled in Parts A and B

Ike began receiving his Social Security cash benefits when he retired at age 62. Since he is already receiving benefits he will automatically be enrolled in Medicare Part A and B the month of his 65th birthday. Approximately 3 months before turning 65, he receives his Medicare card in the mail. Part B premiums will be deducted from his Social Security check beginning the month he turns 65. If Ike does not wish to enroll in Part B at that time, he should indicate that he does not want Part B, return the enclosed notice and no premiums will be deducted from his Social Security check.

Why Should a Person Purchase Part B?

For most people it is advisable to purchase Part B at age 65 because there are penalties for late enrollment and because it is difficult to obtain health insurance coverage in this country for persons over age 65. Persons who do not enroll in Part B at age 65 and who change their minds at a later date face a 10% permanent penalty added to their monthly Part B premium for each year Part B was not purchased. An exception is made for working persons (see next section).

What If a Person Continues to Work Past Age 65?

A person who continues to work past age 65, although eligible for Medicare, can decide to keep his or her employer's group health plan (EGHP) as the *primary* health insurance. This also applies for a 65-year-old person covered by his or her working spouse's plan. Medicare law states that companies with 20 or more employees must offer the same health insurance coverage to employees 65 and older as they offer to younger employees.

Medicare-eligible employees should apply for Part A at age 65, even though they may chose not to receive Social Security cash benefits. They may also decide to defer Part B, for which a monthly premium is charged, until they are no longer covered by the employer group health plan. Employees can defer Part B coverage with no penalty if they choose. Of course, they may also elect to purchase Part B in addition to the company insurance if there are gaps in the employer's plan that Medicare would fill. Medicare will then pay as a "secondary payer" (see "Medicare as a Secondary Payer" in Chapter 6).

A worker 65 and older, whose employer group health plan has ended, can buy Part B *within 7 months after retiring* without incurring the 10% per year penalty. However, it is best to enroll in Medicare during *the month in which you retire because coverage will become effective that month.* The employee should have a letter from the employer stating he or she has just retired. If an employee enrolls after the first month, coverage begins the following month.

If an employee over 65 elects Medicare as his or her *primary* health insurance, then his or her employer may not offer coverage that supplements Medicare. This is obviously meant to discourage employers from shirking their obligation to provide primary coverage.

While still employed, it is up to the employee to select whether Medicare or the company plan will be the primary payer. When the company plan is primary, all claims go to the private carrier first, then to Medicare. If the amount paid by the private insurance is less than what Medicare would have paid as the primary insurance, then Medicare will pay the difference, although this does not happen often. If a retired spouse, age 65, is married to a younger spouse and both are covered by the EGHP, then that plan must be primary for the person age 65. That person may defer Part B with no penalty.

What Does the Medicare Card Look Like?

An example of a Medicare card is shown in Figure 1.1. The claim number is either yours or your spouse's Social Security number (or in the case of a dependent child, it is the parent's). This number is followed by a letter code that is used to identify the type of benefits. When you file a claim, it is important to include the letter codes. (Letter codes are listed in the next section.)

The most common codes are "A," signifying the primary wage earner, and "B," referring to a dependent wife. A dependent husband is a "B1." Often beneficiaries mistake this "A" and "B" designation for their inclusion in Medicare Part A or Part B. Inclusion in Part A and B and enrollment dates are shown at the bottom of the card. Railroad retirees have a letter symbol preceding their claim number.

In 1991 the Health Care Financing Administration will issue new and replacement Medicare cards that specifically state "Hospital (Part A)" and "Medical (Part B)." Cards issued prior to this date identify coverage either as "Hospital Insurance" or "Medical Insurance." In the past many beneficiaries have been confused about whether they were enrolled in "Part A" and "Part B" since this was not stated on the card. Also HCFA will begin adding the word "Medicare" to new and replacement cards and will identify the beneficiary's "Medicare claim number" instead of just the "claim number." Both old and new cards are valid.

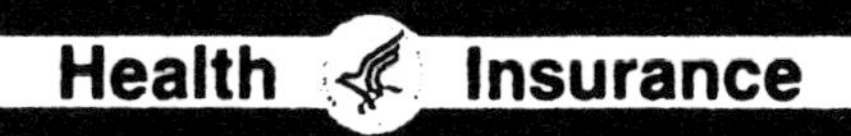

SOCIAL SECURITY ACT

NAME OF BENEFICIARY
HELEN M EVIN

CLAIM NUMBER		SEX
123-34-8025-A		FEMALE
IS ENTITLED TO		EFFECTIVE DATE
HOSPITAL	PART A	7-1-75
MEDICAL	PART B	7-1-75

SIGN
HERE ➡ ______________________

Figure 1.1 Sample Medicare Card

Beneficiary Identification Codes:

- A Retired insurance benefit; person collects benefits on own work record
- B Wife over age 65, receiving benefits from husband's work record
- B1 Husband over age 65, receiving benefits from wife's record
- B6 Divorced wife
- C Child, including disabled adult/child and student
- D Widow
- D1 Widower
- D2 Widow, second claimant
- D6 Surviving divorced wife
- HA Disability insurance benefit
- HB Wife of disabled person
- M Supplemental medical insurance only (Part B)
- W Disabled widow

Railroad Retirement ID Codes That Precede the Social Security Number

- A 123456 Retired railroad employee (a six-digit number is used for persons who retired prior to 1967)
- MA 123456 Spouse of an employe who retired prior to 1967
- A 000-00-0000 Retired railroad employee (social security number is used after 1967)
- MA 000-00-0000 Spouse of railroad retiree
- WA 123-45-6789 Widow or widower of employee who retired before dying
- WD 123-45-6789 Widow or widower of employee who died before retiring

2

MEDICARE PART A

Hospital Insurance

INPATIENT HOSPITAL COVERAGE

What Is Inpatient Hospital Coverage Under Medicare?

Inpatient coverage refers to the services a patient receives after having been admitted to a facility approved by Medicare. Patients who remain in "observation beds," even for overnight stays in the hospital, are not considered inpatients unless they are formally admitted. These days it is no simple matter to admit patients to the hospital.

The Hospital Utilization Review Committees (URC) monitor admissions to ensure that they are appropriate. The care must be "reasonable and necessary" as defined by Medicare. This is determined by the URC, the Medicare intermediary, and the Peer Review Organization (PRO)—a physician-sponsored, nongovernmental organization of health professionals in each state—that maintains a contract with the federal government to review hospital treatment of Medicare patients before, during, and after their stay. (Complaints about quality of care should be directed to your state's Peer Review Organization.)

What Are the Eligibility Requirements for Hospital Admission?

1. The care must be "reasonable and necessary" for a specific disease or illness, as determined by the Utilization Review Committee, the Peer Review Organization (PRO), and the Medicare intermediary.
2. Medicare will reimburse a hospital only if:
   the stay is prescribed by a physician.
   the hospital is the only place where the care could be given.
   the hospital participates in Medicare.
   the stay is approved by the Utilization Review Committee or the Peer Review Committee.

What Are the Basic Inpatient Hospital Benefits Under Medicare?

1. A semiprivate room
2. Meals, including special diets
3. Regular nursing care
4. Special care units, such as coronary care unit, intensive care, etc.

5. Laboratory tests, including outpatient laboratory services performed within 72 hours prior to a hospital admission
6. Drugs given in the hospital
7. Radiology services, such as X rays
8. Medical supplies, such as casts, splints, surgical dressings
9. Use of equipment, such as wheelchairs
10. Blood transfusions (Patients must meet a deductible for the first 3 pints of packed red blood cells, unless blood is replaced; if patients have already paid for the first 3 pints of blood as outpatients under Part B, they will be credited for an inpatient deductible.)
11. Operating room and recovery room costs
12. Rehabilitation services, such as physical therapy, speech therapy, and occupational therapy
13. Medical social services, such as discharge planning
14. Emergency admission to the nearest hospital *without* a physician's order, in life or death situations
15. 190 *lifetime* days in a participating psychiatric hospital
16. Care in participating Christian Science Sanatoriums, if operated or listed and certified by the First Church of Christian Science, Boston

Note: Remember your surgeon, anesthesiologist, hematologist, pathologist, radiologist, pulmonary specialist, family physician, and other physicians are *not* covered under Part A but are covered under Part B.

What Hospital Services Are *Not* Covered by Medicare?

1. Personal convenience items that are requested, such as television, telephone, air conditioner, radio
2. Private duty nursing (Many hospitals discourage the hiring of private duty nurses because it makes record-keeping more difficult.)
3. Extra cost of a private room, unless there is a medical necessity or no semiprivate room is available.
4. Physicians' services (Professional fees that are charged by physicians such as anesthesiologists, radiologists, and pathologists are billed separately under Medicare Part B even though the patient may never meet some of these physicians.)
5. First 3 pints of blood for transfusion
6. Care in a hospital outside the United States (The United States refers to all 50 states, the District of Columbia, Puerto Rico, the Virgin Islands, Guam, American Samoa, the Northern Mariana Islands, and the territorial waters adjoining the land areas of the United States.) If taking a cruise, you should be aware that services rendered aboard a ship in an American port—limited to the same day the ship arrived at or departed from that port—are considered to be rendered in American waters and will be covered. In an emergency or a medically necessary situation, a person may be covered in a Canadian or Mexican hospital, but make sure you get the bill because *you* will have to file the claim. When traveling, Medicare beneficiaries should consider insuring themselves either through their Medicare supplement or through a one-time travel insurance policy.

How Many Hospital Days Are Covered, and What Are the Patient Costs?

Medicare beneficiaries are covered for 90 inpatient days each benefit period. A benefit period begins when the patient enters a hospital and ends when he or she is out of the hospital or a Medicare-approved skilled nursing facility for 60 consecutive days. For the first 60 days in the hospital, Medicare covers all but a specified deductible. In 1991 the deductible is $628. If the patient's hospital stay exceeds 60 days in a benefit period, he or she must pay daily coinsurance. The 1991 daily coinsurance costs for day 61 through day 90 are $157. Patients do have an additional 60 lifetime reserve days (day 91 through day 150), but these days can only be used once and then reserve days are no longer allowed. The patient pays $314 per day coinsurance in 1991 if he or she uses any lifetime reserve days. There is no limit to the number of benefit periods in a person's lifetime. See Table 2.1 for a breakdown of Medicare coverage and benefit days.

The patient pays the hospital only the deductible, plus blood charges and any noncovered services. *The patient is not responsible for charges that exceed Medicare's reimbursement to the hospital.*

If a hospital stay is not approved by Medicare, a patient could be responsible for the hospital charges. The hospital, however, must notify the patient that the charges are not approved, and notification should be given prior to admission. In the event that notification is given during or after a patient's admission, the patient is rarely liable for charges. All Medicare patients should be notified of their appeal rights when they enter a hospital as inpatients.

Who Bills Medicare for a Hospital Stay?

The hospital bills Medicare for a hospital stay. Many patients are upset when they receive the expensive, itemized bills from the hospital after an inpatient stay. Many patients think they owe thousands of dollars, when in fact they will usually be liable only for the deductible. Hospitals should indicate somewhere on the statement if the deductable is due and if Medicare has been billed. The itemized bill *should be checked for errors even though the patient is not responsible for this amount.* Inflated hospital costs result from errors in bookkeeping. In cases where the amount paid by Medicare is less than what the hospital charged, the hospital cannot bill the patient for this additional amount.

How Do Hospitals Get Paid Under Medicare?

In order to get paid by Medicare, hospitals must "participate" in Medicare. Almost all do. (Limited coverage is provided in the few nonparticipating facilities.) Using a standard UB-82 form, hospitals bill the Medicare intermediary. Medicare reimburses the hospital directly. The patient receives a record of this payment in the form of a Medicare Benefit Notice.

What Are the Prospective Payment System and the Diagnosis Related Groups, and How Do They Affect How Hospitals Are Paid by Medicare?

Before the new Prospective Payment System was put in place in 1983 to curb escalating costs, hospitals were reimbursed based on reasonable costs. The longer the stay and the more services performed, the more the hospital was paid.

Under the Prospective Payment System, hospitalized Medicare patient illness and surgery are classified into 490 Diagnosis Related Groups (DRGs). Hospitals are reimbursed a predetermined, fixed amount for a specific DRG that is assigned to the patient at discharge, even though the amount the hospital billed (the actual charge) is often more than what the hospital is reimbursed by Medicare under the DRGs. Because the fixed reimbursement amount is based on the patient's primary diagnosis, and *not on the length of stay* or *actual cost,* hospitals have a financial incentive to discharge patients earlier.

Certain hospitals such as psychiatric, rehabilitation, and cancer hospitals are not reimbursed under the DRG system, even though Medicare will cover approved services. Also excluded are hospitals outside the 50 states (Washington, D.C. and Puerto Rico come under the DRG system), and those hospitals that are reimbursed under special arrangement.

Rumor has it that hospitals are discharging Medicare patients "quicker and sicker" these days. There is conflicting evidence as to whether or not these shorter hospital stays are in the long run detrimental to a patient's health. If you are ever told that your Medicare days are used up and that is the reason you are being discharged early, it is not true.

Patients who feel they are being discharged prematurely may request a written explanation of the noncoverage from the hospital and may start an appeal proceeding. The hospital's patient representative or a trained Medicare advocate can assist in this process (see Appeals in Chapter 5).

SKILLED NURSING FACILITY COVERAGE

What Is Skilled Nursing Facility Care, and Does Medicare Cover this Kind of Care?

Skilled nursing care does *not* refer to the type of long-term care most people associate with nursing homes. According to the Medicare definition, skilled care is a level of care that is provided under the direction of a physician or other licensed professional, such as a registered nurse, licensed practical nurse, physical therapist or speech pathologist, and that includes treatments for inpatients who have illnesses or injuries that seriously affect their life or health.

Under the Medicare guidelines, Medicare covers only a small portion of inpatient skilled nursing care costs and only if this care is provided in a Medicare-certified skilled nursing facility. (Skilled nursing facility [SNF] coverage is also called "extended care.") To be eligible for SNF coverage, you must occupy a Medicare-certified bed in a licensed "skilled" nursing home or in a hospital.

Not all nursing homes are licensed as skilled, and of those, not all have "Medicare-certified" beds. For example, for some rural hospitals with less than 99 beds, a special certification is issued allowing the hospital to use a certain number of beds as both inpatient beds and skilled nursing facility beds. These are called "swing beds."

The intent of SNF coverage is to address acute situations that can be cured, restored to a former condition, or improved by short-term *daily* care or rehabilitation. In reality, only a small percentage of the population qualifies for SNF benefits. Intermediate, custodial, and rest home care are not covered.

To confuse matters, there are conditions that ordinarily do not require skilled services but may require them under some circumstances. For example, taking blood pressure does not ordinarily require a skilled professional and is usually considered custodial care, but an unstable patient recovering from heart surgery and taking a new medication may require a skilled nurse to monitor blood pressure. This may then be covered under the Part A SNF benefit.

How Does a Person Qualify for Skilled Nursing Facility Care?

1. The physician must certify that the patient needs, actually receives, and will benefit from skilled nursing care and/or skilled rehabilitation services on a daily basis.

   Skilled nursing services include:

   technical services, such as tube feeding, Foley insertion, open wound care/dressing, decubitus care, post-cataract care, and intravenous administration.

   observation and assessment of a medically unstable patient (one at risk of deteriorating in the immediate future), such as a patient who is at risk from possible dehydration and who is being considered for tube feeding or a patient whose response to a medication must be monitored.

   patient instruction in the self-care of devices, such as newly established ostomies, tracheotomy tubes, indwelling catheters; instruction in diabetic care, gastrostomy feeding, or self-injections.

   Rehabilitative services consist of:

   physical therapy services including evaluation, transfer training, therapeutic exercise, gait training, electrotherapy, prosthetic training, muscle re-education, etc.

   occupational therapy services including evaluations, daily living skills training, perceptual motor training, sensory treatment, fine motor coordination, etc.

   speech therapy services including evaluation, voice disorders treatment, speech articulation disorders treatment, aural rehabilitation, dysphagia treatment, etc.
2. Under these circumstances, services can only be provided in an SNF on an inpatient basis.
3. Service must be reasonable and necessary and consistent with medical opinion.
4. The stay cannot be disapproved by Peer Review Organization or the facility's Utilization Review Committee.
5. The facility must be a Medicare-certified, skilled nursing facility that has the staff and equipment to provide skilled nursing, rehabilitation, and other health services.
6. The patient must have been hospitalized for 3 consecutive days prior to admission and must be admitted within 30 days of hospital discharge.

Note: Services that are not skilled include administration of routine oral medications or eye drops; general maintenance care of colostomy or ileostomy; changing of nonsterile dressings, general methods of caring for incontinent patients, etc.

What Are the Basic Skilled Nursing Facility Benefits?

1. A maximum of 100 days per benefit period with 3 days prior hospitalization required
2. A semiprivate room
3. Meals, including special diets
4. Regular nursing care
5. Rehabilitation services that include physical, speech, and occupational therapy (If you receive therapy, but not every day, therapy services may be billed under Part B and not included under Part A coverage.)
6. Drugs administered in the facility
7. Medical supplies including splints and casts
8. Equipment such as oxygen and wheelchairs (Some SNFs lease equipment to inpatients.)
9. Blood, after a patient pays for the first 3 pints

Note: Again, as in the hospital, the physician's visits are covered under Part B of Medicare and are not included as a Part A benefit.

What Skilled Nursing Facility Services Are *Not* Covered by Medicare Benefits?

1. Personal convenience items, such as television and telephone

2. Private duty nursing
3. Private room, unless it is medically necessary
4. Physician's services (For Medicare-approved SNF stays, the physician is reimbursed under Part B for seeing a new patient upon arrival and then for two visits the first week and one visit each week thereafter.)
5. First 3 pints of blood
6. Intermediate or custodial care (Even though the patient's family thinks the patient may need "skilled care," Medicare has the final say. Of course, the patient may appeal. If a Medicare beneficiary *is* a resident of a nursing home and is not receiving skilled care, Medicare Part B covers patient visits by physician/physician assistant/nurse practitioner team at the rate of one-and-one-half visits per month. Other Part B services may also be covered, although Medicare will not cover room and board. Interestingly, oxygen is not covered by Medicare for a patient who lives in a nursing home although it is a benefit for a person living at home who requires oxygen.)

What Is the Maximum Number of Skilled Nursing Facility Days a Person Is Entitled to, and What Are the Costs?

In 1991 a beneficiary is entitled to a total of 100 Medicare-approved days in a Medicare-certified skilled nursing facility. There is a 3-day prior hospitalization requirement to be eligible. This 3-day stay does not include the day of discharge. For the first 20 days, there is no patient coinsurance; however, from day 21 through day 100, the patient is responsible for a daily coinsurance amount of $78.50. There may be other noncovered charges that are also the patient's responsibility. (See Table 2.1 for a breakdown of Medicare coverage and benefit days.)

Who Bills Medicare for a Skilled Nursing Facility Stay?

The skilled nursing facility will bill the Medicare Part A intermediary for all approved services, and Medicare will reimburse the facility directly. Costs are covered in full *except* for coinsurance, noncovered services, or services that are billable under Part B of Medicare, such as physician visits. The patient will receive a record of the claims in the form of a Medicare Benefit Notice.

TABLE 2.1 Part A Medicare Coverage (Based on 1991 Figures*)

Inpatient Hospital Coverage	**Medicare pays**
Days 1 through 60 in a benefit period	all but $628 deductible
Days 61 through 90 in a benefit period	all but $157 per day
Days 90 through 150 in a benefit period (these 60 days are lifetime reserve days)	all but $314 per day
After 150 days in a benefit period	nothing
Skilled Nursing Facility Benefit	
Days 1 through 20 in a benefit period	all
Days 21 through 100 in a benefit period	all but $78.50 per day
Over 100 days	nothing
Home Health Care	
Up to 35 hours per week or short-term daily care up to 21 days	all eligible expenses and 80% of durable medical equipment
Hospice Benefit	
210 lifetime days that can be extended with physician's certification	all but 5% of cost of drugs and respite care (maximum $628)

*Figures change annually.

HOME HEALTH CARE COVERAGE

What Is Home Health Care?

When ill, many people prefer to remain in their own homes and may require in-home services such as personal care, health care, or housekeeping assistance. Home health care can be considered a part of the continuum of long-term care. The long-term care continuum consists of a wide range of services and living arrangements including housekeeping services, adult day care, live-in companions, live-in nurses, assisted living facilities, and/or nursing homes. Medicare pays for only a small portion of costs in this continuum.

People are often confused about the qualifications for home health care, the type of care provided, and the period of time covered. Medicare pays for home care only if the type of care needed is skilled and is required on a part-time or intermittent basis. Home care is intended to help people recover or improve from an illness; not to provide unskilled services over a long period of time. However, intermediaries must evaluate each case disregarding whether the patient's condition is chronic or stable. Intermediaries cannot deny a patient home care benefits simply because the patient is not expected to improve rapidly.

When Is a Person Eligible for Home Health Care Benefits?

1. A patient must be homebound, that is, not able to leave the home without physical assistance from another person or special equipment such as a wheelchair or a walker.
2. A patient must require skilled care by a registered nurse or licensed practical nurse, physical therapist or speech therapist.
3. A physician must certify that the care is reasonable and medically necessary for the documented diagnosis and must develop a plan of care.
4. The care must be required on an intermittent or part-time basis.
5. The services must be provided by a "participating" home health agency.

What Are Some Common Diagnoses that May Require Skilled Home Health Care?

It is the physician who must decide that the following diagnoses require skilled home health care according to Medicare's guidelines. Remember that sometimes unskilled services may be deemed skilled. For example, administering eye drops normally is an unskilled task; however, it may require a skilled professional for a Parkinson's disease patient who has had cataract surgery. The following list includes some of the common diagnoses that necessitate skilled care by a home health agency.

Fractures
Cardiac disease
Stroke
Diabetes
Post-surgical complications
Complications of respiratory diseases
Complications of cancer

What Are the Basic Home Health Care Benefits?

1. Part-time skilled nursing (A registered nurse or licensed practical nurse must open the case even though this first visit is not paid by Medicare.)
2. Part-time physical therapist
3. Part-time speech therapist
4. If the patient is receiving any of the above services, *then* the following services may also be provided:

   Occupational therapy, which includes assistance in regaining the skills of daily living, such as combing hair, toileting, feeding, etc.

   Part-time services of a home health aide that are provided under the supervision of a skilled nurse or physician (The home health aide usually provides services three times per week for about 2 hours each time. The aide must spend approximately 80% of the time performing personal care services such as helping with walking, eating, bathing, and shaving, and the other 20% performing duties such as grocery shopping, housekeeping, etc.)

   Medical social services provided by a medical social worker who assists with placement in an institution or plans ongoing medical care after Medicare no longer pays for home health care

   Medical supplies, such as bandages, incontinence pads, lamb's wool pads, catheters, irrigating kits, sheets, ostomy bags, syringes, casts (The agency should bill Medicare for supplies.)

   Durable medical equipment used repeatedly and rented or purchased from a medical equipment supplier (*Medicare only covers 80% of an approved charge* for medical equipment such as wheelchairs, hemodialysis equipment (no coinsurance charged), semi-electric hospital bed, respirators, crutches, quad canes, reach bars, walkers, nebulizers, suction machines, bedside commodes, oxygen and oxygen equipment and tents, and, in some cases, water mattresses and heat lamps. The home health agency often assists the patient with rental or purchase information.)

Note: Noncovered medical equipment includes air conditioners, humidifiers, posture chairs, safety grab bars and bathroom equipment.

What Is *Not* Covered as Part of Home Health Care?

1. Blood transfusions
2. Full-time nursing

3. Homemaker services including nonmedical support services such as grocery shopping, food preparation
4. Drugs and biologicals (Only the procedure and the skilled professional are covered by Medicare, not the actual pills, insulin, antigens, serums, vaccines.)
5. Meals delivered to the home
6. Transportation to and from a covered service that is not available in the home
7. The 20% Medicare-approved charge for durable medical equipment, plus any amount above an approved charge

How Long Can a Beneficiary Receive Home Health Care Benefits, and What Are the Costs?

In theory, a beneficiary who requires skilled care at least once every 60 days is eligible for home health services. Careful and appropriate documentation by the home health agency is really the key to getting the services one requires. As a general rule, part-time home health care is covered up to and including 28 hours a week for any number of days for less than 8 hours a day and on a case-by-case basis, and up to 35 hours a week for less than 8 hours a day if deemed reasonable and necessary. Intermittent care is provided up to and including 28 hours a week *on a less than daily basis,* and up to 35 hours per week on a less than daily basis if deemed reasonable and necessary. In some circumstances, a patient can receive short-term daily care up to 8 hours per day for a maximum of 21 consecutive days, or longer in certain circumstances (see Table 2.1 for a breakdown of home health care coverage).

Medicare pays the full amount that has been approved for all covered home health visits. There are no patient coinsurance, annual deductible, or number of visit limitations. The patient, however, does have to pay 20% of the Medicare-approved charge for any durable medical equipment.

Who Bills Medicare for Home Health Care?

All home health care claims are submitted by the home health agency to Medicare. Payment goes directly to the provider of services. The supplier is responsible for billing Medicare for durable medical equipment. Services provided by the physical and speech therapists are billed through the home health agency.

HOSPICE CARE COVERAGE

What Is Hospice Care?

Hospice care was added to Medicare in 1982 and became effective in 1983. The purpose of hospice care is to provide in-home (nonhospital) care for symptom management, pain relief, and support services to persons certified by a physician to be terminally ill and not expected to live beyond 6 months. A terminally ill patient may voluntarily choose hospice care in lieu of regular Medicare services. However, there must be a responsible person who can give or coordinate the patient's care in the home. It is important to remember that patients who elect hospice care forfeit their right to use the Medicare system in the standard way and instead must have all care for their terminal illness managed by the hospice program. (Conditions *not* related to the terminal illness are billed to Medicare in the standard way.) At any time the patient can reject hospice care and reapply for regular Medicare services.

What Is a Hospice?

Medicare defines a hospice as "a public agency or private organization that is primarily engaged in providing pain relief, symptom management, and supportive services to terminally ill people and their families." These agencies are similar to home health agencies, except services are directed toward the needs of the terminally ill patient. A hospice must have a certification from Medicare before it can provide hospice services.

Some communities have inpatient hospice facilities. Some of these have Medicare certification, others do not. Hospices in the community are generally private-pay facilities that may be licensed by the state as nursing homes or hospitals. They employ professionals who are trained in serving the needs of terminally ill patients.

Who Provides Hospice Care?

Care is generally provided by a Medicare-certified hospice agency. The hospice agency manages services related to terminal illness and provides appropriate professional staff, pain-relief medicines, supplies, etc. to the person *in the home.* The Medicare health maintenance organizations may offer their enrollees other options concerning where they receive hospice care.

What Does Hospice Care Include?

1. Physician services
2. Nursing (registered nurse or licensed practical nurse)
3. Drugs (Under the hospice benefit, Medicare covers any drug related to the primary diagnosis to relieve symptoms, such as drugs to relieve pain, nausea, constipation, or anxiety; and, in some cases, antibiotics. Chemotherapy agents are not covered.)
4. Physical, speech, and occupational therapy
5. Home health aides
6. Homemaker services
7. Medical social services, including social workers
8. Medical supplies and appliances
9. *Short-term* inpatient care, including *respite* stays (see section below) in a hospital or skilled nursing facility.
10. Counseling, including family counselors, chaplains, support groups

What Is Respite Care?

Only under the hospice benefit does Medicare cover limited "respite care." Medicare defines respite care as "a short-term inpatient stay in a nursing home or hospital, which may be necessary for the patient in order to give temporary relief to the person who regularly assists with home care. Inpatient respite care is limited to stays of no more than 5 days in a row." How often a person is approved for respite stays is determined on a case-by-case basis. To emphasize, the purpose of respite care is to provide the *caregiver*, not the patient, a respite from the day-to-day responsibilities of caring for an ill family member or friend.

How Long Is a Person Eligible for Hospice Care?

A person is entitled to 210 lifetime days of hospice care; however, this limit can be extended if the person is recertified as terminally ill at the end of the period (see Table 2.1). Hospice care is divided into benefit periods. The first and second benefit periods consist of 90 days each, and the third consists of 30 days. If patients decide to end hospice care once a benefit period is under way, they must forfeit the remaining days but only in that benefit period. Thus if patients who are in day 10 of their second 90-day benefit period decide to end hospice care, they permanently forfeit 80 days. They can resume hospice care but it will begin in the third and last benefit period, which has a total of 30 days, although care now can be extended indefinitely if the person is still terminally ill. Of course, patients can revert to the standard Medicare services at any time.

A Medicare hospice must continue care if the patient requires and requests it. The patient, however, can be billed by the hospice agency for this continued care.

Who Bills Medicare for Hospice Care?

The hospice agency bills Medicare (this includes inpatient hospital claims). The patient's physician continues to bill Medicare Part B directly.

What Are the Patient's Costs?

Medicare pays for all covered services. The patient pays 5% of the reasonable cost of drugs or $5 per prescription, whichever is less, and 5% of the cost of respite care (about $4 to $5/day), not to exceed the Part A hospital deductible. Medicare-certified inpatient hospices may charge a Medicare patient a daily amount to cover the cost of room and board.

3

MEDICARE PART B

Medical Insurance

OUTPATIENT SERVICES

What Is Medicare Part B (Also Called Medical Insurance)?

Medicare Part B covers outpatient treatments, as well as physicans' services whether inpatient or outpatient. Outpatient services are services provided to patients who are not "admitted" to a hospital, a skilled nursing facility, or other inpatient facility.

Does Medicare Pay for Part B Expenses the Same as for Part A?

No, the Part B payment system is different from Part A. Part B requires an annual deductible ($100 in 1991), then Medicare pays 80% of a Medicare-approved charge. (How the approved charge is calculated is discussed later in this chapter.) Medicare beneficiaries are responsible for paying coinsurance equal to 20% of the Medicare-approved charge and for any amount over the Medicare-approved charge ("excess") if the service provider *does not accept Medicare assignment,* plus charges for services not covered by Part B.

What Are the Medicare Beneficiary's Costs Under Part B?

The Part B Medicare plan is voluntary and has a monthly premium, which is usually deducted from a person's Social Security check. Persons who do not receive monthly cash benefits from Social Security but who are enrolled in Part B are billed for Medicare by the government. In 1991, a person enrolled in Part B pays a monthly premium of $29.90. In addition to the monthly premium, there are also beneficiary costs that include

- an annual $100 deductible.
- the 20% Medicare-approved charges.
- amounts in excess of Medicare-approved charges on unassigned claims.
- the first 3 pints of blood for transfusion.
- noncovered services.

Who Bills Medicare for Part B Claims?

Before September 1, 1990, claims for Part B were submitted to Medicare by the Medicare beneficiary, the physician (or other providers of services), a hospital, or any other institution billing for a Part B covered service. Since September 1, 1990, all service providers are required to submit Part B claims for beneficiaries.

How Does a Beneficiary Keep Track of Part B Claims?

When Medicare pays a claim either directly to a provider or to the beneficiary, the beneficiary receives an Explanation Of Medicare Benefits (EOMB). The EOMB is a statement describing who provided the services, when the services were provided, what services were rendered, whether the Medicare assignment was accepted, the actual charges billed to Medicare, what amount was approved by Medicare, and how much Medicare paid on the claim. It also keeps track of the beneficiary's annual deductible. The EOMB is *not* a bill; it is merely a statement describing the facts relating to a claim.

What Are the Eligibility Requirements for Receiving Services Under Part B?

1. The person must be enrolled in Part B of Medicare.
2. The care received must be "reasonable and necessary in the diagnosis and treatment of a specific illness or injury." This is determined by the physician and the Medicare carrier. Medicare does not cover preventive or routine care. A person must be ill or injured before Medicare pays. For example, Medicare does not cover a routine eye exam for eyeglasses, but it will cover eye care for a patient with glaucoma.

What Physician Services Does Part B Cover?

A physician is defined as a medical doctor (M.D.). This includes psychiatrists,* psychologists,* osteopaths (D.O.), dental surgeons,* chiropractors,* optometrists,* and podiatrists.* (Part B coverage is limited for starred (*) providers.) Medicare covers the following professional services:

1. Surgical services, including anesthesia (The following surgeries must have pre-admission approval from the Peer Review Organization.)
   - Bunionectomy
   - Cataract procedures
   - Carotid endarterectomy
   - Coronary artery bypass graft
   - Percutaneous transluminal coronary angioplasty (Medicare has been denying the "standby" services of a cardiac surgeon during this procedure although many hospitals require that the surgeon be available. This policy may be challenged in the future.)
   - Permanent pacemaker
   - Bypass graft-vein
   - Hysterectomy
   - Laminectomy
   - Major joint replacement
2. Medical services
3. Services provided by physician's nurses and staff
4. Physician charges (professional component) for the interpretation of diagnostic tests and procedures such as electroencephalogram (EEG), X rays, basal metabolism rate, upper GI series, blood tests, urine analysis, bone scans, CAT scans, angiograms, myelograms, X-ray and radioactive isotope therapy, pathological services, and chemotherapy, etc.

Note: Effective January 1, 1992, physicians will be prohibited from billing Medicare or the patient for interpretation of electrocardiograms (EKGs) as a separate item when it is provided as part of a physician visit or consultation.

5. Transfusions of blood and blood components
6. Drugs and biologicals that cannot be self-administered (insulin is not included)
7. Therapies that are planned and reviewed by a physician, including physical therapy, occupational therapy, and speech pathology services

These therapies must be medically necessary and may be received in a physician's office or from an independently practicing Medicare-certified therapist (occupational or physical therapy only, no speech therapy) in the therapist's office or the beneficiary's home. In 1991 Medicare will approve a maximum of $750 and pay 80% of that amount or $600/year. Patient may also recieve therapy as an outpatient of a participating hospital, a skilled nursing facility, a home health agency, clinic rehabilitation agency, or public health agency approved by Medicare (no dollar limit).

Note: Remember if physical therapy, occupational therapy, or speech therpay is provided as part of an inpatient stay or as part of the home health benefit, the patient has no coinsurance responsiblity.

8. Medical supplies

9. Second opinion regarding surgery

If you cannot find a physician, you can call a toll-free Medicare second opinion referral center (1-800-638-6833; in Maryland 1-800-492-6603) for the names and telephone numbers of physicians in your area who will provide a second opinion.

10. Clinical laboratory diagnostic services—diagnostic clinical laboratory tests provided by independent laboratories or by physicians must be submitted to Medicare as assigned claims

Medicare will pay 100% of a Medicare-approved amount, and the patient pays no coinsurance. A patient should not be billed for most diagnostic clinical laboratory tests, such as blood tests, urinalysis, cultures, pro times, etc.

11. Mental illness services—limited

Medicare Part B will help pay for limited psychiatric evaluations (including testing), medication consultations, and outpatient treatment of mental illness. Services must be billed by a psychiatrist, a psychologist employed by the psychiatrist, a clinical psychologist who accepts assignment, a clinical social worker employed by an outpatient mental health center that accepts assignment, a physician's assistant employed by a physician, or a comprehensive outpatient rehabilitation center (CORF). Claims for therapeutic services are paid at 50% of the approved charge, except for hospital outpatient treatment and diagnostic services that are not subject to this limit.

Note: Organic brain syndrome is not considered a mental illness by Medicare.

12. Chiropractor's services—limited

Medicare normally covers 12 visits per year for subluxation treatment (partial or incomplete dislocation of spine) if condition is shown on an X ray. Part B will not pay for the chiropractor to take X rays, provide heat treatments, give ultrasound, or do physical therapy.

13. Podiatrist's services—limited

Only injuries and diseases of the foot are covered. Generally, one visit every 60 days for treatments such as debridement (removing dead tissue) of mycotic (fungal) toenails, or removal of plantar (foot sole) warts is covered. Cutting toenails, treatment of corns, callouses, and flat feet are not covered. Bunionectomy is covered if prior approval has been obtained from the Peer Review Organization.

14. Optometrist's services—limited

Eye exams, performed by an optometrist who is legally authorized by the state, for disease or injury, and replacement of organic lens with contact lenses or eyeglasses after cataract surgery are covered. Medicare will help pay for one pair of conventional eyeglasses or contact lenses following cataract surgery for insertion of an intraocular lens. If the cataract has been removed and no intraocular lens has been inserted, however, the provider can submit bills for eyeglass lenses and frames to Medicare once a year if medically necessary. Medicare does *not* pay for refractions (eye exams that measure the eye for eyeglasses).

15. Dental surgeon's sevices—limited

This covers surgery of the jaw or related structures, fractures of the jaw or facial bones, or diseases—such as cancer—that would be covered if treated by a physician. Implants and buildup of the alveolar ridge (teeth ridge) due to bone loss caused by prior biting or chewing problems are *not* covered. Generally, there is only a slight chance that dental problems will be covered. An *inpatient hospital stay for a severe dental procedure may be covered,* even though the dental surgeon's service would not be covered.

What Outpatient Hospital Services Are Covered by Part B?

When a Medicare beneficiary is diagnosed and treated for an illness or injury in a Medicare participating hospital, the outpatient services listed below are covered. (For purists reading this book, these services are actually billed to the Medicare Part A "intermediary" rather than to the Part B "carrier," even though they are Part B benefits.)

1. Diagnostic tests and clinical laboratory tests billed by the hospital (Medicare pays 100% of clinical laboratory tests.)
2. Services in the emergency room or an outpatient clinic
3. X rays and other radiological services, such as radiation therapy
4. Medical supplies, such as gauze, ointments, bandages (including ace bandages), splints, and casts
5. Drugs and biologicals that cannot be self-administered
6. Blood transfusions

Under Part B, the patient must pay for the first 3 pints of blood each year unless the blood is replaced or unless this deductible was already paid for under Part A.

7. Outpatient surgical services

Part B helps to pay for specified outpatient surgical procedures in a Medicare-certified "Ambulatory Surgical Center" (ASC), which can be hospital-affiliated or independent. The ASC must have an agreement with Medicare and must only perform outpatient surgery services.

8. Kidney dialysis

What Other Miscellaneous Services Are Covered by Part B?

1. Ambulance service is covered in cases of emergency or accident or when other transport would endanger the patient's health. Service to and from a local hospital or a skilled nursing facility is usually covered. In cases where a patient has chest pain, is unconscious, or needs telemetry (continuous monitoring of the heart), an ambulance must take the patient to the nearest emergency room unless there is an Intensive Care Unit (ICU) divert at that hospital, meaning the hospital cannot take the patient in the ICU. In cases where there is a medical necessity requiring ambulance service, Medicare will help cover ambulance charges *from* a nursing home *to* a hospital *to* a nursing home—for example, if a patient is having a nasogastric tube replaced. Ambulance rates depend on whether the person receives basic life support or advanced life support. Medicare does not cover an Amb-o-cab. Air ambulance transport is covered if the point of pickup is inaccessible by land vehicle, is remote, or if the patient might not survive if transported by land.
2. Portable diagnostic X-ray services are covered when they are received at home or in a nursing home and if they are ordered by a physician and supplied by a Medicare-certified supplier.
3. Equipment and supplies are covered if they are prescribed by a physician and obtained from a Medicare-certified supplier.

   Durable medical equipment (DME). Refers to medically necessary, reusable items that are prescribed by a physician and are used in the home for a specific illness or injury. Medicare will cover equipment if a patient has a physician's prescription and gives this to the medical supplier before renting or purchasing equipment. Covered items include oxygen and oxygen equipment (coverage is determined by the percentage of oxygen saturation in the blood), wheelchairs, some traction equipment, hemodialysis equipment, respirators, crutches, canes, walkers, TENS units (electrical nerve stimulation to relieve pain), hospital beds, seat lift chairs (only the mechanism is covered, not the chair), electric wheelchairs, nebulizers, suction machines, and, in some cases, a water mattress and commodes (if patient is 100% bedridden). Noncovered medical equipment includes air conditioners, humidifiers, posture chairs, safety grab bars, and bathroom equipment.

Medicare classifies durable medical equipment into the following categories:

Inexpensive or other routinely purchased DME. These items are billed to Medicare as purchased items; their price cannot exceed $150 (includes commodes, walkers, and crutches).

Items requiring frequent and substantial servicing. Medicare makes rental payments on these items until the medical necessity ends (includes ventilators and dialysis equipment).

Customized items. These are billed to Medicare as purchased items only (includes specially constructed wheelchairs).

Other prosthetic and orthotic devices. These devices are billed to Medicare as purchased items only (includes artificial limbs; excludes intraocular lenses).

Capped rental items. Rental payments are made by Medicare for up to 15 months of continuous use (includes standard wheelchair, hospital beds).

Oxygen and Oxygen equipment. Medicare pays on a monthly basis according to a fee schedule (includes liquid, gaseous, or concentrator systems). Nebulizers are included in this category.

Medicare pays monthly rental fees for DME. The amount of the monthly rental payment is either the lowest actual charge for the equipment or an amount determined by Medicare's fee schedule. The monthly payments are initially 10% of an area's "recognized purchase price." Medicare will only pay for up to 15 months of continuous use. If medical need for the equipment exceeds 15 months, Medicare will make a maintenance and servicing payment during the first month of each succeeding 6-month period.

Home oxygen equipment is paid on a monthly fee schedule determined by liter flow. A physician's certification is required every 12 months certifying a patient's need for oxygen. Under Part B, oxygen is not covered for persons living in a nursing home, since a nursing home is not considered a person's residence. However, oxygen is covered under the Part A SNF benefit for persons receiving oxygen in a nursing home.

Prosthetic Devices. Devices that replace a body part or a malfunctioning body part, such as artificial limbs and eyes, urinary incontinence supplies (not diapers or sheets), corneal implant, ostomy bags and supplies are prosthetic devices. Also covered are orthotics (rigid or semi-rigid joint or muscle braces) such as cervical collars, molded knee joints, and orthopedic shoes (only if they are part of a leg brace). Arch supports, elastic stockings, and molded shoes are not covered. Medicare limits its annual payments on ostomy and urinary incontinence supplies. Note: Included as part of the Part A Home Health Benefit are catheters, catheter supplies, ostomy bags and ostomy care supplies.

Medical Supplies. These include surgical dressings, lamb's wool pads, catheters, irrigating kits, splints, and casts but not common first aid supplies.

4. Home health care is billed under Part B when patients are not enrolled in Part A of Medicare, but it only covers 80% of the allowable charges. A person receiving physical or occupational therapy or speech pathology services in the home from a Medicare-certified home health agency is responsible for the $100 deductible and 20% coinsurance.
5. Comprehensive outpatient rehabilitation facility (CORF) claims must be "assigned". This is strictly an outpatient coverage and includes physician services; physical, speech, occupational, and respiratory services; counseling, etc.
6. Screening PAP tests are covered every 3 years or more frequently for high-risk patients.
7. Injectable drugs for treatment of osteoporosis for homebound patients unable to administer the drugs themselves are approved for treatment of bone fractures related to postmenopausal osteoporosis.
8. Screening mammography including preventive X ray and the physician's interpretation is covered every 24 months for women age 65 and older (may cover more often for high risk patients).

Will Medicare Pay for Outpatient Prescription Drugs?

No, but there is an exception. Medicare does cover 80% of an approved charge for immunosuppressive drugs but only during the first year following a Medicare-covered organ transplant. Also, biologicals such as hemophilia blood clotting factor and antigens (substance that stimulates the body to produce an antibody) are covered in medically necessary circumstances.

What Outpatient and Physician Services Are *Not* Covered by Part B?

1. Prescription drugs
2. Homemaker services (such as shopping, cleaning, companionship)
3. Foreign health care

There are exceptions. If you need inpatient *emergency* care, or nonemergency inpatient care and a Mexican or Canadian facility is the closest facility available, Medicare may help pay. Physician and ambulance service may also be covered in these situations.

4. Meals on Wheels
5. Personal convenience items
6. Services performed by immediate family
7. Services that are custodial in nature
8. Items or services that the Veterans Administration provides free of charge or that are payable by Workers Compensation, automobile, travel liability insurance, employer health plans, or other governmental programs
9. Routine physicals and tests they entail
10. Routine eye exams for glasses and the eyeglasses; all refractions
11. Routine hearing tests and hearing aids
12. Routine foot care, such as cutting toenails, treatment of corns, callouses, and flat feet
13. Routine immunizations, except pneumonia vaccination (no coinsurance charged); Hepatitis B vaccine for high-risk persons; immunizations required to treat immediate risk of infection, such as from tetanus; and

influenza vaccine covered during flu season through the first part of 1992 and only in certain areas of the country

14. Cosmetic surgery unless it is required because of accidental injury or to improve a malformation
15. Routine dental care, including dentures, fillings, cleaning, surgery for impacted teeth, and other surgery involving structures supporting the teeth
16. Alcohol or drug dependency treatment
17. Acupuncture
18. Services connected with experimental medical procedures, considered "not medically necessary"
19. Administration of drugs that can be self-administered, such as insulin. (Exceptions are chemotherapy agents and injectable drugs for osteoporosis.)
20. Services of a Christian Science practitioner or naturopath.

How Do Part B Claims Get Paid?

For Part B services, Medicare pays 80% of a charge that it considers reasonable. This reasonable charge is called the Medicare "approved" or Medicare "allowed" charge. It is often lower than what the provider actually billed. The Part B claim is filed to the Medicare carrier as either an assigned or unassigned claim. How the claim is classified affects how much the beneficiary will ultimately have to pay. All providers are required to send claims to Medicare on behalf of their patients.

Note: Medicare beneficiaries should be aware that in the case of elective surgery (surgery that is not an emergency), the surgeon and the assisting surgeon who do not accept assignment *must notify the patient in writing* before surgery of the approximate amount the patient will have to pay out-of-pocket if the cost of the surgery is $500 or more. If notification is not given, the physician must refund any payment of the "excess" made by the patient. Anesthesiologists are presently exempt.

Unassigned Claims

The total amount the provider charges the patient is called the "actual charge." Some providers do not "accept Medicare assignment," so when the bill for the actual charge goes to Medicare, it is said to be "unassigned." On an unassigned claim, providers expect to get paid the actual charge for their service. Medicare may pay some of the charge, but the patient is expected to pay 20% of the approved charge as coinsurance plus the "excess," which is the difference between what Medicare approved and the actual charge (see Table 3.1). Actual charges are limited by the government for Medicare services

EXAMPLE

Dr. Gim Mee charged Corona $75 for a recent visit to his office. Corona paid the physician with a check. The physician's office filed a claim to Medicare. Several weeks later Medicare sent Corona an Explanation of Medicare Benefits and a check for $48. Medicare had received the claim for the $75 actual charge and determined that $60 was the Medicare "allowable" or "approved" charge for that service. Since Part B claims are reimbursed at 80% of the Medicare "approved" charge, Medicare multiplied $.80 \times \$60 = \$48.00$ and sent a check for $48 to Corona. Corona had now been reimbursed $48 of the $75 she had paid to Dr. Mee. She had no other insurance to bill, so her "out-of-pocket" expense for that visit was $27.

Assigned Claims

If providers agree to "accept Medicare assignment," their bills are sent to Medicare and are said to be "assigned." On an assigned claim, the provider, even though billing Medicare for the actual charge, usually does not get paid that amount. When a claim is assigned,

Medicare must mail the payment directly to the provider instead of the patient, because the patient has "assigned payment" to the provider, and

providers accept the "Medicare-approved amount" as the maximum amount they will charge the patient.

Providers must "write off" any amount over and above the Medicare-approved amount. They cannot bill the patient for the "excess" amount, which is called "balance billing" (see Table 3.1).

EXAMPLE

Dr. Ike Cept's bill for Corona's visit was $75. Dr. Cept's office sent the claim to Medicare. Several weeks later, Dr. Cept's office received a payment from Medicare for Corona's claim. Medicare had approved $60 and had sent the physician $48. Because Dr. Cept had agreed to accept assignment and, therefore, had agreed not to charge Corona any more than what Medicare approved, he subtracted $48 from $60 and billed Corona for $12. Since Corona did not have any other insurance, her out-of-pocket expense for that visit totaled only $12.

TABLE 3.1 Comparison of Unassigned and Assigned Claims

Types of Charges/Payments	Unassigned Claims	*Assigned Claims*
Physican charge	$75	$75
Medicare-approved charge	$60	$60
Medicare payment of 80% of approved charge	$48	$48
Coinsurance payment	$12*	$12*
Excess	$15*	**

* What Corona Pays.
** Not applicable for unassigned claims.

Does Medicare Limit a Person's Out-of-Pocket Expenses?

No, Medicare does not limit a person's out-of-pocket expenses..

How Does Medicare Arrive at Its "Approved" Payment Amount?

Medicare uses "fee screens" to arrive at its reasonable or "approved" amount. Because this information is at least a year or two old, the approved charge will usually be lower than the provider's actual charge. The Medicare "approved" or "allowed" amount will be the lowest of any one of the following charges:

1. The physician's actual charge for the service
2. The physician's customary charge, that is, the median charge for the service to the physician's Medicare patients during the past year
3. The prevailing charge in the geographical region, that is, a customary charge for services based on an established percentile level for all physicians in a particular region

Despite the fact that Medicare is a uniform federal program, physicians have traditionally been paid different amounts, depending on where they practiced. Between 1984 and 1986, there was also a national fee freeze. Nonparticipating providers could not raise their actual charges for Medicare patients during that time. In January 1987, they were allowed to raise actual charges but only within the federal "increase limits." Nonparticipating providers are still feeling the negative effects—although the fee freeze ended in 1986—since they are locked into a lower prevailing charge.

Are Health Care Providers Required to Give Information on Living Wills?

The Omnibus Budget Reconciliation Act of 1990 (OBRA 1990) requires Medicare and Medicaid health service providers to maintain written policies and procedures related to living wills and advance directives. Under state law, providers are required to give written information to all adult patients about their rights regarding medical care decisions; providers also must inquire whether a person has an advance directive and they cannot discriminate against those that do; they must ensure compliance with state law concerning advance directives; and they must educate their staff on advance directives.

How Do You Know if a Provider Accepts Medicare Assignment?

Physicians who "participate" in Medicare sign a contract with Medicare agreeing *always* to accept Medicare assignment for Medicare patients. In 1989, 37.8% of physicians, other medical practitioners, and suppliers participated in Medicare.

Nonparticipating physicians, although they do not formally "participate" in Medicare, sometimes agree to accept assignment on an individual basis. If, for example, a person is having financial difficulty or cannot afford more than an inexpensive Medicare supplement, he or she may want to ask the provider to accept assignment. Or, if there is a period of illness that incurred a lot of medical bills, a person may ask the physician to accept assignment for a specified period of time. A handful of states (Massachusetts, Pennsylvania, Connecticut, Vermont, Rhode Island) have enacted different regulations mandating Medicare assignment.

What Is the Maximum Allowable Actual Charge?

Through December 1990, the maximum allowable actual charge (MAAC) limited the amounts nonparticipating providers could charge Medicare patients for their services. A nonparticipating physician's actual charge for a particular service could not exceed his or her MAAC, which is determined, like it or not, by Medicare. Each year Medicare notifies physicians of their MAACs, which are determined by comparing a participating physician's actual charge for services with a percentage of the current prevailing charges of nonparticipating physicians and using whichever is lower. In 1991 nonparticipating physicians' charges are capped by a "limiting charge" (see next section).

Are There Reforms in Physician Payment on the Horizon?

In November 1989 Congress passed a "physician payment reform" bill that attempts to make Medicare fees more equitable for physicians and to halt rising health care costs. There are three main features of the bill: national fee schedule, limits on the amount physician charge, and limits on volume of service.

National Fee Schedule

Beginning in 1992, and to be phased in over five years, Medicare will reimburse physicians according to the lesser of actual charges or a "national fee schedule" based on a "resource based relative value scale" (RBRVS). The fee schedule for nonparticipating physicians will be 95% of the amount payable to participating physicians. The Health Care Financing Administration supported a study of the RBRVS by a group of researchers from Harvard, under the direction of William Hsiao, Ph.D. The goal was to reform and make more equitable the reimbursements to physicians under Medicare. Historically, family practitioners, for example, have been compensated at much lower amounts than specialists. Our system has rewarded high technology and provided a disincentive to primary care physicians who often spend more time with their patients. The RBRVS is a nonmonetary scale that would have to be multiplied by a dollar amount. The scale presently identifies values for 1,400 medical procedures and ranks them, taking the following into consideration.

1. The amount of work a physician performs on a certain service, including time before, during, and after the service and the intensity with which the time is spent
2. Practice costs, such as office expenses, salaries, etc.
3. A malpractice component that reflects the portion of a physician's resources that is spent on malpractice expenses

Limits on the Amount Physicians Can Charge

Beginning in 1991, physicians who do not accept assignment can charge Medicare patients a maximum of 125% (140% on certain physician evaluation and management procedures) of the Medicare-aproved amount. This upper-limit allowance is called the "limiting charge."

Limits on Volume of Services

By limiting the rate by which Medicare Part B spending can increase beyond a projected amount each year, this measure reduces physicians' annual payment beyond that rate. In other words, if services exceed the Medicare Volume Performance Standard (MVPS) for the year, the inflation increase in the fee schedule will be reduced the next year.

4

FILLING MEDICARE GAPS

SUPPLEMENTAL INSURANCE OPTIONS

What Are the Options for Supplementing Medicare?

Medicare does not cover an older person's health care costs entirely, nor was it designed to do so. Medicare covers between 40% and 50% of a person's health care costs. Part A of Medicare does a good job of covering an inpatient hospital stay, which would otherwise be very expensive, but does not do a good job covering long-term nursing home or home health care. Because Part B of Medicare only covers one third of the personal health care costs for physician and outpatient services, most Americans choose to supplement Medicare with one or more of the following options.

- Purchase a Medicare supplemental insurance policy
- Continue or convert employer group insurance
- Join a health maintenance organization (HMO)
- Purchase long-term care insurance
- Purchase indemnity benefits insurance policies, such as hospital insurance, "dread disease" insurance, and accident policies
- Apply for Medicaid, if eligible
- Use veterans or retired military benefits, if eligible
- Pay out of their own pocket

How Do You Decide Whether to Supplement Medicare?

Present good health should not be the only factor in determining whether or not you will need to buy supplemental health insurance in the future, since health can change. You must decide whether you have the funds and are willing to cover the dollar amounts not paid by Medicare for deductibles, prescription drugs, portions of physician's services, and other eventualities. Most people seek some form of supplemental insurance. They buy insurance and hope they will not need it but are reassured by the fact that it will be there if they do.

Consider whether you have the option of receiving or purchasing health benefits from former employment, whether it be civil service, military service, or a large corporation. If so, find out *exactly* how you will be covered and how much it will cost. What are the chances that one day insurance coverage will not be available? Talk to other retirees who have filed claims with the plan you are investigating. *Not all employer-sponsored group health plans for retirees are the best choice.* They are not regulated by state insurance departments. Many have a lot of fancy language but very poor coverage. In the case of retired military personnel who use military facilities, the wait for services may be long. In addition, not all routine and specialized care may be covered. Some insurance plans may not be guaranteed renewable, benefits could change over the years, or the company could go out of business and disband the group.

If you are a low-income Medicare beneficiary, you should investigate whether you are eligible for Medicaid (see Medicaid, Chapter 8).

If you decide you do need to purchase a supplement, you must decide whether to purchase an individual or group insurance policy or become a member of a health maintenance organization (HMO). Contact health maintenance organizations in your area and discuss their coverage and rates.

Far more difficult and confusing is the selection of an appropriate insurance policy from a private insurer since there are so many companies and so many policies. Seek out qualified senior health insurance counseling programs in your area. A number of states, including Colorado, Washington, California, and Massachusetts, have programs to assist older adults with issues of health insurance, including policy comparisons. They will not recommend policies, but they can help you interpret some of the policies you are considering.

If no counseling services are available

a. ask friends who have filed many claims and are satisfied with the way their policies pay on claims.
b. ask the bookkeeper in your physician's office, or in a hospital's accounting office, which companies pay promptly.
c. meet with insurance agents or brokers to gather information or perhaps with a few friends (start with agents you or your friends know).
d. find out if your state's Commissioner of Insurance has a shopper's guide that lists the insurance options.

What Are the Medicare Gaps (Medigaps) That Need to Be Supplemented?

Before making decisions about how to supplement Medicare, you should be familiar with Medicare's gaps (what Medicare does not cover) including deductibles, coinsurance, excess charges, and noncovered services. Familiarize yourself with the following list because, ideally, you are looking for insurance to cover as many of these areas as you need and can afford. It is very important to understand what you are buying since duplication of coverage is costly and wasteful. For 1991, Medicare does *not* cover the areas listed below.

Medicare Part A Gaps

- Hospital deductible per benefit period = $628
- Hospital coinsurance per benefit period for days 61 to 90 = $157 per day
- Hospital coinsurance per benefit period for days 91 to 150 = $314 per day
- No coverage for inpatient psychiatric care after 190 lifetime days are used
- Skilled nursing facility coinsurance per benefit period for days 21 to 100 = $78.50 per day
- Any nursing home care other than Medicare's 100 skilled days (Costs may range from $50 per day in rural areas to $150 per day in urban areas.)
- Home health care coinsurance for durable medical equipment = 20% of an approved charge plus expenses for any home care that is not skilled or is not covered by Medicare; home health aide and homemaker services ($10 – $12/hour and up); private duty nursing ($26/hour and up for registered nurse and $18/hour and up for licensed practical nurse—minimum 2 hours on average)
- Hospice coinsurance for respite care (maximum $628) and drug coinsurance (up to $5 per prescription)

Part B Gaps

- Annual $100 deductible
- The 20% coinsurance on Medicare-approved charges
- Amounts in excess of Medicare-approved charges

Additional Gaps

- First 3 pints of blood
- Prescription and nonprescription drugs
- Medical expenses while traveling abroad
- Any care, whether inpatient or outpatient, that is not "reasonable and necessary"
- Routine care, such as physicals, eye exams, eyeglasses ($100 – $250 + per pair), hearing tests, hearing aids

($250 + used, $425 + new), dental exams, dentures ($450 - $1,000)

- Preventive or wellness services
- Equipment that is considered nonmedical or custodial
- Physical therapy/speech pathology $30 - 40/hour average) that is not covered under Medicare's stringent definitions

MEDIGAP INSURANCE

What Is Medicare Supplemental (or Medigap) Insurance?

Many Americans supplement Medicare by buying special insurance policies to help cover Medicare deductibles, coinsurance amounts, and noncovered benefits. There are a number of companies selling these policies, offering a wide range of prices for policies and benefits. Medicare supplements generally pay a percentage of the cost of services, rather than a fixed daily dollar amount.

In 1982 minimum federal requirements were established for Medicare supplemental policies (Baucus Amendment, 1981). Policies meeting these standards are said to be "certified." Most states have passed laws adopting these requirements in order to certify Medicare supplements sold in that state. Some of the minimum requirements are listed below.

1. Policy must disclose the benefits of the policy in an easy-to-read format.
2. Company must have a "loss ratio" of at least 60% on individual policies (new legislation will raise this to 65%) and at least 75% on group policies. This means the company must pay out in claims at least 60% to 75% of the money it collects from premiums over the life of the policy.
3. Policyholder must have the right to cancel and obtain *full* refund on a policy up to 30 days after delivery of policy.
4. Policy cannot add a rider that excludes policyholder from coverage at a later date.

Because there is little federal regulation of the insurance industry in this country, the National Association of Insurance Commissioners (NAIC) sets policy by designing model regulations that then can be adopted by individual states. Laws adopted by the states must be at least as stringent as the NAIC model for Medicare supplements. Otherwise, the Health Care Financing Administration is charged with "certifying" each Medicare supplement in that state, something most states do not relish.

From time to time Congress instructs the NAIC to revise the model regulations for minimum benefit standards for Medicare supplemental policies. Most states adopt the NAIC model and, subsequently, pass their own legislation establishing minimum benefits. Some states legislate stricter minimum standards for policies sold in that state.

In addition to the above minimum requirements, certified Medicare supplements must also

a. cover either all or none of Medicare Part A $628 deductible.
b. cover the hospital coinsurance for days 61-90 (at $157 per day) and for days 91-150 (at $314 per day).
c. pay 90% of an additional 365 days if lifetime reserve days (days 91-150) are used up.
d. cover the blood deductible under Part A or B, unless the blood is replaced.
e. cover *at least* 20% of Medicare-approved Part B coinsurance after a maximum annual deductible of $100.
f. guarantee renewability for individual and group policies.
g. eliminate waiting periods for preexisting conditions on replacement policies.
h. cover preexisting conditions after a maximum waiting period of 6 months.

The Omnibus Budget Reconciliation Act of 1990 (OBRA 1990) gives the NAIC 9 months to develop a uniform language and format on policies marketed as Medicare supplemental insurance; the same period of time is given to develop up to 10 standard Medigap packages. This act prohibits the sale of a Medigap policy to persons who already hold policies and intend to keep them or who are eligible for Medicaid. It increases the loss ratios for individual policies from 60 to 65% and requires refunds if loss ratios are not met. It requires a 6-month ban on medical underwriting when a person age 65 or older first enrolls in Medicare Part B. Most states will pass legislation based on these model regulations.

Note: Remember to check with your State Insurance Division for 1991 Medicare supplemental regulations that apply to your state.

What Would the "Ideal" Medicare Supplement Include?

Policies that are called "Medicare supplements" generally pay only for Medicare-covered services and only after Medicare pays first. If Medicare denies payment for a service, the supplemental policy will not pay.

Most insurance experts agree that a person needs only one Medicare supplement, and yet some figures show that 25% of dollars spent for Medicare supplements are spent on unnecessary or overlapping coverage.

As a starting place, we have designed an ideal Medicare supplemental policy that would cover important Medicare gaps. No such policy exists, but we can dream! An ideal Medicare supplemental insurance policy would include the following:

1. It covers Part A hospital deductible and all hospital coinsurance.
2. It covers the coinsurance in a skilled nursing facility (SNF) for days 21–100.
3. It covers an extra 265 days of skilled care per year and 365 days of intermediate or custodial care in any state-licensed nursing home. (This would not be contingent on exhausting Medicare SNF benefit days.)
4. It covers the Medicare Part B deductible.
5. It covers all Part B Medicare eligible expenses up to what the provider actually charges. (Until every provider always accepts Medicare "assignment," this coverage should be part of the policy.)
6. It covers the blood deductible, whether incurred under Part A or Part B.
7. It covers 80% of prescription drugs after a $100 deductible.
8. It covers medical expenses while traveling abroad.
9. It covers one routine physical exam per year.
10. It covers 80% of the cost of eyeglasses, dentures, and hearing aids.
11. It guarantees a renewable policy for life.
12. The premiums do not increase with policyholder's age.
13. The policy is in full force immediately; no waiting period for preexisting conditions.
14. It cannot exclude a person because of health conditions; provides "guaranteed issue".
15. It is available to disabled Medicare beneficiaries under age 65.
16. It is insured by a company that is financial stable and always in business.
17. Claims will be automatically filed to supplemental company.
18. The policy does not cost more than $75 per month.

How Do You Find a Good Medicare Supplement?

1. Determine an affordable price range. The average cost of a Medicare supplement is about $60–$65 per month.
2. Review Medicare's gaps and determine which ones are most important for your individual needs. For example, some people do not need to buy a policy that covers *all* of the Part B excess charges.
3. Work with companies and/or licensed agents you know, whenever possible.
4. Talk with friends who have been ill and are satisfied with their insurance and have had a lot of good claims experiences.
5. Look into supplements offered by senior associations and professional groups. But be careful, they may or may not be less expensive. Some companies form "senior associations" just to get you to buy their insurance. Also, policies issued before the 1990 regulations took effect may not offer the guaranteed renewability you seek. Check with your state's insurance division.
6. Call the State Insurance Commissioner's office to get a list of policies certified for sale in your state or consult a consumer shopper's guide, if available. You can also check if a company is in good standing, but it is hard to get the "real scoop" on a company. No one with integrity can guarantee that a company will always be there for you, no matter how long they have been in business.
7. Ask if the premiums increase with policyholder's age. No increase is best.
8. Ask if a physical exam or a physician's report is required in order to apply for the policy (called "health underwriting"). If so, answer everything honestly and completely.
9. Read carefully all the provisions for renewing the policy, especially if your policy was issued before 1990. It is best to have a guaranteed renewable or noncancelable policy. The following lists the different types of renewal conditions found in insurance policies:

   No provisions for renewal.

   Renewable at the option of the company. The company usually selects a certain term, such as the policy anniversary date, to determine whether it will renew your policy.

   Conditionally renewable. The insured person has the right to continue the policy in force by timely payments of premiums; the insurer cannot make a change in any provision of the policy but can change premiums on a class basis (such as all people of a certain age or gender) and can decide not to renew by class, by geographic area, or other stated reasons other than age or deterioration of health.

Guaranteed renewable. The insured person has the right to continue the policy in force by timely payments of premiums; the insurer cannot change the terms of the policy or cannot decline to renew but may change the premium if it is changed for all persons of a particular class (such as all policyholders of a certain state or age). Most Medicare supplements are guaranteed renewable for life. Keep in mind that if your policy is with a group and is guaranteed renewable and if the group is terminated, so is your policy. (This may not be applicable to some policies issued after 1990.) Also, companies do go out of business! Does your state have a "guaranty fund" to protect you if this happens?

Noncancelable. This is a *continuous* term policy that cannot be canceled and cannot raise premiums. It is hard to find this language.

Cancelable. This policy can be terminated by either the insured or the company if 30-days notice is given.

10. Ask what kind of riders are available and how much you must pay. Riders may cover extra benefits, such as services not covered by Medicare.
11. Ask if the agent will be available to service the policy after selling it to you. Find out how long he or she has worked in the present office. An agent generally makes his or her largest commission from the first year of sale. The commission can be as high as 50% of your policy premium. Some states are attempting to pass laws to regulate agent commissions; however, these laws are being challenged.
12. Ask what the company's *A. M. Best Insurance Reports* rating is and how long they have been in business? The A. M. Best Company is an independent analyst of the insurance industry. (A company must subscribe to get a rating.) The company reviews the financial status of thousands of insurers and assigns ratings that reflect the relative financial strength and operating performance of companies and compares these to the accepted norms of the industry. Ratings change, however, and policies should not be selected solely on the basis of this rating. An A+ (superior) is the highest rating, followed by A (excellent), B+ (very good), B (good), C+ (fairly good), C (fair). Young companies, companies that do not subscribe to A. M. Best, and nonprofit health, hospital, and medical service corporations are not rated.
13. Avoid duplicating coverage. Purchase one good policy. There is an exception. In a few cases only, you might want to hold on to a second policy, such as a policy through former employment that provides special benefits (like prescription drugs) or a policy through the federal government. You may not be able to repurchase this type of policy at a later date if you cancel. As an example, consider the widower who dropped his federal benefits when he and his wife became eligible for Medicaid. After his wife died, the widower sold his house and because of the income he received from the sale, he lost his Medicaid coverage and had to purchase a new Medicare supplement. He could not repurchase the federal benefits he had canceled.
14. Since there are laws prohibiting waiting periods for preexisting conditions, when replacing one Medigap policy with another, you should not have to overlap policies when purchasing a new one.
15. Benefits *must be written* to be valid, despite what an agent may say. If it sounds like gobbledygook it probably is. Do not wait until you submit a claim to review your policy.
16. Shy away from agents—and their policies— who give you a deadline to buy.
17. Pay by check only, made payable to the company and not the agent.
18. Do not buy policies that are made to appear as if they are offered by the government, often emblazoned with red, white, and blue symbols, eagles, etc. This practice is against the law.
18. Stick with your current policy if it provides good coverage.
19. Review your policy every year with a qualified person to make sure it is up-to-date and competitively priced.

Can the Premiums for Medicare Supplements Be Considered an Itemized Tax Deduction?

Yes.

What Are Some of the Advantages of Medicare Supplemental Policies?

1. Policyholders have free choice of physicians and hospitals.
2. A person can select a policy that covers those Medigaps determined to be important to his or her individual needs.
3. Most policyholders are covered anywhere in the United States.

What Are Some of the Disadvantages of Medicare Supplemental Policies?

1. Comprehensive policies are expensive and may be denied to people with health problems.
2. Unless the policyholder has a very comprehensive policy, he or she may not be able to project out-of-pocket costs.
3. The policyholder must file claims and manage medical billing paperwork.
4. The policy language may be hard to understand.

EMPLOYER GROUP HEALTH PLANS

Are Employer Group Health Plans a Good Way to Supplement Medicare?

Some employers offer retired employees health insurance that will supplement Medicare when the retiree reaches age 65. Many retired people are covered by employer group plans. Often the coverage is good, offering additional benefits that Medicare does not pay; and because it is a group plan, the premiums are often less expensive. The retiree may not have to pay premiums or may be asked to pay for part or all of the premiums out of a retirement or pension plan.

Some company retirement health benefits continue to offer the same benefits as when the person was employed. However, now the plan coordinates those benefits with Medicare, paying only after Medicare pays. To determine benefits the company calculates what it would have paid if the plan paid first and then subtracts whatever Medicare has paid. These are known as "carve-out" policies. They are not technically "Medicare supplements" and are not subject to state Medicare supplemental regulations. It is often *very* difficult to determine from employee manuals just exactly how these policies work in terms of dollars and cents, because the section on retiree benefits is usually very short and often written by people who don't understand how Medicare works. It is best to find a company benefits adviser who is knowledgeable about Medicare and who can explain the way the company's plan pays.

Sometimes employees are offered an opportunity to convert their prior group health insurance to a Medicare supplemental policy with the same insurer. Generally there is no new health underwriting or waiting period, but this policy could cost more and offer less.

Not all employer group plans are better than policies purchased in the marketplace, so it is wise to evaluate and compare. Also consider the security of the company plan and whether premium costs have gone up regularly and will continue to go up. Over time employer group health plans, including privately funded plans, may decrease benefits, increase premiums, or go bankrupt.

What Is COBRA Continuation Coverage?

The Consolidated Omnibus Budget Reconciliation Act (1986), commonly referred to as COBRA, provides continuation of employer-provided health coverage for persons who would otherwise lose this benefit. COBRA can assist people who upon retirement lose their employer-provided health benefits. These retirees have a difficult, if not impossible, time purchasing health insurance. Under the COBRA continuation option the law requires certain employers to allow "qualified beneficiaries" whose group health insurance would otherwise end to purchase continued coverage at the group premium rate (plus up to 2% extra for administration) for up to 3 years. An employer who maintains a group health plan (including a self-insured plan) and employs 20 or more employees must offer this option. Religious organizations and the federal government are not covered by COBRA although state and local governments are covered. If a company goes out of business or if the employer ends health coverage for all employees, the COBRA continuation option *does not apply.*

A "qualified beneficiary" refers to employees, including former and retired employees, their spouses, and dependent children. Should a qualified employee lose group health insurance coverage because he or she is fired, quits, retires, has work hours reduced, is involved in strikes or walkouts, or takes maternity/paternity leave, the employee can elect to purchase continuation of his or her health plan under the COBRA law. Termination of employment for reasons of gross misconduct or layoffs does not entitle a person to COBRA continuation. The COBRA option is available to the spouse and dependents if the covered employee dies, loses employment for reasons other than gross misconduct, has work hours reduced, becomes eligible for Medicare, or divorces or separates from a spouse.

COBRA coverage generally lasts for up to 18 months if employment was terminated for any reason other than gross misconduct or reduced hours. If a second "qualifying event" occurs in the 18-month period—for example, the death of the covered employee during this period—the spouse and dependent children may be entitled to an additional 18-month extension up to a total of 36 months. As a result of legislation effective in 1990, disabled employees who are eligible for Social Security disability at the time of termination of employment have the option of continuing coverage under COBRA for 29 months, instead of 18 months.

To continue coverage, the employee must make timely premium payments. Premiums cannot exceed 102% of the group rate, except for disabled persons, in which case premiums can go up to 15% of the group rate for the 18th through the 29th month. Some states require a group health plan to offer the qualifying employee the option to convert to an individual policy after the continuation period is up. However, the premiums are often prohibitive!

HEALTH MAINTENANCE ORGANIZATION PLANS

What Are Health Maintenance Organizations (HMOs)?

Health maintenance organizations (HMOs) are systems of "managed care" that provide direct medical services to persons living in a defined geographic area in return for a prepaid fixed monthly premium and often a small fixed copayment at the time of each service. Think of them as your insurance company and your medical provider rolled into one. HMO enrollees must use specified health care providers (physicians, hospitals, skilled nursing facilities, medical equipment suppliers, etc.).

Medicare beneficiaries who enroll in HMOs or competitive medical plans (CMPs) are still responsible for the Part B premium. Medicare-contracting HMOs and CMPs often cover preventive services not covered by traditional health insurance or Medicare. Medicare beneficiaries cannot be denied for health reasons a standard membership in an HMO that has a *risk contract* with Medicare. However, enrollees must meet the following requirements.

- Live within the covered area of the HMO
- Pay the HMO monthly premium (if there is one)
- Be enrolled in Part B of Medicare (Persons who have Part B only and do not have Part A will pay a higher monthly premium.)
- Apply for HMO membership (Contract HMOs must have at least one 30-day enrollment period each year.)
- Not have end-stage renal disease
- Not be in a hospice-election period

Persons may stay enrolled in an HMO regardless of health if the above conditions are met. If the HMO ends its contract with Medicare, memberships are canceled, and the Medicare beneficiary will be given at least 60-days notice. If beneficiaries are inpatients during this period, their coverage will continue until discharge.

What Are the Basic Types of HMOs?

Staff Model

Physician and staff are employed by the HMO and care is provided at the HMO's facility.

Group Model

A group of physicians contract with an HMO to provide care at centrally located sites.

Individual Practice Association (IPA)

Individual physicians in private practice contract with an HMO to provide services in their offices.

Preferred Provider Organization (PPO)

This is a variation of an HMO that is primarily offered to insured employee groups. (In some states standard Medicare beneficiaries may be eligible to join.) The PPO physicians and providers furnish services to members for lower than usual fees in return for prompt payment and a certain volume of patients. Members may see a physician outside the PPO list, but they will pay deductibles and coinsurance. If PPO members choose a provider from the group's list of PPO providers, they often receive full first-dollar coverage.

What Are the Types of HMO Affiliations That Work with Medicare?

Noncontract HMO

Under this type of HMO plan, the Medicare beneficiary pays a monthly fee to receive medical care from a specific group of providers affiliated with the HMO. The HMO bills Medicare for "reasonable costs" of services provided. The patient does not pay Medicare deductibles or coinsurance if he or she uses the HMO providers. The patient, however, does pay the Medicare Part B monthly premium, a monthly premium to the HMO (if there is one), and a fixed copayment at the time of each visit (if this is required by the HMO).

The patient can seek care from non-HMO providers in the community, and Medicare can be billed by these non-HMO providers for eligible expenses. However, the patient is then responsible for the usual Medicare deductibles and coinsurance. In other words, the patient has a financial incentive to use the services of the HMO to which he or she belongs.

Contract HMO

Under this type of plan, the HMO enters into a contract with the federal government. The HMO agrees to provide enrollees with at least all Part B benefits that are covered by Medicare. In return, the government agrees to pay a specific fixed amount to the HMO each month for each Medicare beneficiary who is enrolled. The Health Care Financing Administration (HCFA) negotiates payment arrangements with the HMO depending on whether the contract is a "cost"—including a hybrid known as health care prepayment plans (HCPP)—or "risk" contract:

Cost contract. The HMO is paid by the HCFA based on the cost of taking care of each patient, in addition to a minimal payment per month for each enrollee. Unlike risk contracts, these plans are not reimbursed by the HCFA for services not covered by Medicare. The patient pays a monthly premium (if any) and a copayment at the time of each medical visit. The enrollee has a financial incentive to use the services of the HMO since this limits out-of-pocket expenses and eliminates claim filing. The enrollee can use a non-HMO provider, and Medicare will pay its share. However, Medicare deductibles and coinsurance will be the patient's responsibility.

HCPP contracts are similar to "cost" contracts. However, HCPPs are paid by the HCFA for Part B services. The HCPPs do not automatically cover Part A deductibles and coinsurance as do the HMOs' cost and risk contract. Also, they are allowed to underwrite, so they may deny coverage to a person with a preexisting medical condition.

Risk contract. Medicare pays a predetermined fixed monthly amount to the HMO for each enrollee, and the HMO accepts the financial risk of providing care for this fixed payment. If Medicare beneficiaries meet the qualifications previously listed in this chapter, they cannot be refused enrollment for preexisting medical conditions. Risk contract HMOs have a "lock-in" feature, which means that if the patient goes to a physician or provider who is *not* part of the HMO, *neither Medicare, nor the HMO* will pay anything. Emergency situations and authorized referrals are the exceptions. The patient pays a monthly premium, if any, and a copayment at the time of a medical visit. The HCFA is encouraging this type of Medicare HMO in the belief that it controls costs, although in late 1990 there were just under 100 risk contract HMOs/CMPs with approximately 1,000,000 enrollees.

The enrolled Medicare beneficiary must still pay the Part B premiums, plus any monthly premium charged by the HMO and any specified copayments at the time of service.

Can Beneficiaries Disenroll from an HMO?

Yes. They must notify the HMO *in writing* at least one month before they wish to disenroll. The HMO will notify Medicare and, hopefully, within one month the Medicare computer will show the beneficiary as disenrolled and free to use non-HMO providers.

However, there have been delays with disenrollment. Sometimes months go by before Medicare shows that the person is back in the standard Medicare system. During this time, the patient must use the HMO and claims filed to Medicare are consistently denied (although Medicare is ultimately responsible). If this should happen, be persistent in reinstating your "standard" Medicare.

Are the Monthly Premiums for HMOs an Itemized Tax Deduction?

Yes.

As a Medicare Beneficiary, What Are the Advantages of Joining an HMO?

1. Monthly membership premiums cover all Part A and Part B deductibles and coinsurance amounts. Patients may be required to make only a small copayment at the time of a medical visit, which gives patients a realistic idea of out-of-pocket expenses.
2. In addition to standard Medicare benefits, HMOs often provide extra benefits, such as eye exams, regular checkups, prescription drugs, etc.
3. The Medicare beneficiary cannot be denied standard memberships for health reasons in a Medicare HMO, with the previously noted exceptions.
4. All services including day and night emergency services must be provided promptly.
5. HMOs have a financial incentive to provide preventive care.
6. HMO members have no paperwork, no forms or claims to file, and no problems with the "accepting assignment" provision.
7. HMO care is coordinated by a primary care physician; many services are often available in one facility.

What Are the Disadvantages of an HMO?

1. Patients must use providers and facilities designated by the HMO ("lock-in" feature) and may have to give up long-time relationships with their own doctors.
2. Patients are not covered outside the HMO service area (emergencies and urgent care are exceptions, but the patient must attempt to get approval first).
3. Patients may not always be able to see their primary care physician, and they may sometimes receive routine care from a physician's assistant and nurse practitioner instead of an M.D.
4. The HMOs operate within a strict budget, and health care is delivered in as efficient a manner as possible. This means unnecessary tests, extra visits, and routine referrals to specialists may be avoided. This may or may not be a problem.
5. An HMO may cancel its contract with Medicare. If this occurs, the enrollee must be given 60-days notice.

How Can a Person Determine a Quality HMO?

1. Are all the doctors board-certified? Ask for their board specialties.
2. How long does it usually take to get an appointment with the primary care specialist? Ask other patients.
3. In addition to the usual Medicare benefits, what extra benefits are provided?
4. Does the HMO use a good hospital?
5. In emergency situations, will the HMO give you a difficult time if you have to be transported to a non-HMO hospital or use non-HMO physicians? Must you call the HMO first?
6. If malpractice is suspected, must you first submit to binding arbitration with the HMO?
7. How is the quality of the health care service monitored?
8. Is the HMO financially stable? (This may not be easy to find out.)

INDEMNITY AND OTHER LIMITED POLICIES

What Are "Indemnity" and Other "Limited" Policies?

Indemnity policies pay a specific dollar amount to the policyholder, regardless of actual charges, when certain conditions are met. They are not tied into Medicare benefits. The dollar amount is decided when the policy is purchased and remains the same in future years. For example, a "hospital benefits" policy may specify a payment of $30 per day to the policyholder beginning on day 5 of a hospitalization and also may specify an additional $10 per day if the person is confined to an intensive care unit. These policies generally do not coordinate benefits with other insurance policies, that is, they will pay the specified benefits even when another company is paying benefits. *Indemnity policies are not recommended as supplements to Medicare.*

Some types of insurance pay for specific diseases, such as cancer. These policies are nicknamed "dread disease" policies and pay up to a certain dollar amount to the patient according to a predetermined fee schedule. Dread disease policies generally will not pay if another health insurance is paying for the treatment. *Dread disease policies are not recommended by the experts and are illegal in some states.*

Accident policies also pay based on fee schedules printed in the policy. It may be difficult to collect if there is a question, for example, whether a fall has been caused by an accident or by a medical condition such as osteoporosis. Incidentally, in the event of an accident, Medicare is not the primary or first payer if the person who was at fault has liability insurance, no-fault insurance, or a self-insurance plan.

Medicare beneficiaries should consider purchasing a comprehensive Medicare supplemental policy or joining an HMO before purchasing any other type of policy. Because Medicare plus a good supplement will cover most of a person's hospital expenses, the types of policies previously discussed may be useful only for incidental expenses.

LONG-TERM CARE INSURANCE PLANS

What Is Long-Term Care, and How Does a Medicare Beneficiary Insure Against the Catastrophic Expenses of Long-Term Care?

Long-term care describes a continuum of care that is required by a chronically ill or aged person over a period of time. It does not merely refer to care in a nursing home. A person's need for services varies over a period of time and that need usually increases with age or as an illness progresses. The type of long-term care required varies from person to person. A person may need adult day care or part-time or full-time home support services such as homemakers, delivered meals, or home nursing care. Or the person may need the personal care provided by a boarding home or an assisted living facility. Patients recovering from an acute illness may need to live temporarily in a nursing home; still others, unable to care for themselves, may need the custodial care provided by a nursing home.

At present, there are not many options for protecting yourself from the catastrophic expenses of long-term care, whether that care be in the home or in an alternative living arrangement, including a nursing home. Although the Medicare skilled nursing facility (SNF) benefit and home health care (HHC) benefit pay for some short-term skilled nursing care, they are not designed to provide the type of long-term custodial care most people need. In fact, according to Health Care Financing Administration figures, in 1989 Medicare paid only 8% of the nation's $47.9 billion nursing home care bill while out-of-pocket expenditures accounted for 44% of the total cost. Medicaid contributed 43%, private health insurance paid for 1%, and the remaining 4% was covered by Veterans Affairs and other sources.

Financing long-term care is an issue being studied by many groups, including the federal government. Some groups recommend extending Medicare benefits to cover long-term care. The main drawback to having Medicare pay for the costs of long-term care is the financial burden it will create. At present, the options of paying for long-term care in the United States include private pay or Medicaid. Private pay includes payment from personal income, savings, reverse mortgages, home equity conversions, long-term care insurance, and/or life insurance to cover nursing home expenses. Medicaid is discussed in Chapter 8.

The cost of nursing home care in 1989 varied from $25,000 to $50,000 per year or about $2,000 to $4,100 per month. Nursing home care averaged between $2,100 and $2,400 per month. The cost of home care in 1989 averaged $5,000 per year for three visits per week from a home health aide.

What Is Long-Term Care Insurance?

Long-term care insurance is the "new kid on the block" in the insurance industry and has only begun to be marketed by the insurance industry in the last few years. Over 100 companies now sell these products. Traditionally, these policies were unregulated, limited in the benefits they provided, and expensive. According to a recent study conducted by the United Seniors Health Cooperative in Washington, D.C., a person who purchased a nursing home policy in 1988 would have 4 chances out of 10 of ever collecting on coverage. As interest in these products increases, however, new policies are being modified and states are beginning to regulate benefits. It is estimated that about 1 million Americans now have long-term care policies. If you purchased a policy more than a year ago, review your benefits after reading this section.

As one insurance broker stated, "long-term care insurance is an asset protection policy." Careful consideration should be given to the purchase of long-term care insurance. Some of the literature suggests that if a person's income is under $15,000 and assets or savings below $30,000 (excluding a home), long-term care insurance is probably *not* a reasonable option.

What Variables Should Be Considered When Shopping for Long-Term Care Insurance?

When shopping for long-term care insurance, there are many benefit choices. Better coverage, however, means a more expensive policy. The National Association of Insurance Commissioners (NAIC) provides recommended minimum standards for state regulatory programs; these standards are intended to help protect consumers. At its December 1990 meeting, the NAIC adopted a package of consumer amendments to its Long-Term Care Insurance Model Act and Regulation. Under the amendments, all individual policies are guaranteed renewable, and when policies are removed from the market or taken over by a new carrier (as in a group policy), policyholders receive similar benefits as in the old policy. Written disclosures explaining whether the applicant already has a long-term care policy and whether a policy is being replaced are required in the Model Act. The Act specifically prohibits the practice of "twisting," in which an agent sells a replacement policy simply to earn a higher commission. New waiting periods are also prohibited on replacement policies.

To learn what laws are in effect in your state, contact your state's Insurance Division. Remember that individual states enact their own regulations based on the NAIC's Model Act.

The following is a list of the options to consider when purchasing a long-term care policy.

What Levels of Care Does the Policy Cover?

Most policies now cover skilled, intermediate, and custodial levels of care in both state-licensed skilled nursing facilities and intermediate care facilities. Some policies may have stricter requirements for facility licensing. Many policies add limited home health care or convalescent care benefits. Some policies include adult day care or respite care. The following definitions clarify the different levels of care.

Skilled. Nursing or rehabilitative services are available 24 hours a day and are administered by skilled personnel, such as a registered nurse, physical therapist, speech pathologist, or medical doctor. This kind of care restores a patient to a former level of health. Care must be based on a physician's orders.

Intermediate. Occasional care is provided by skilled nursing or rehabilitation professionals and is combined with personal care. Care requires fewer skilled procedures and is based on physician's orders.

Custodial. Services do not necessarily require skilled nursing care, instead services provide personal assistance in the activities of daily living (ADLs) including eating, dressing, toileting, bathing, and moving about. These services can be performed by a nonmedically trained person. In a nursing home, services might include administering oral medications, changing nonsterile dressings, or turning patients who are bedridden. Care is usually based on a physician's certification or opinion that care is necessary.

Home care. Services range from skilled to nonmedical and are provided at home. (Presently this is a grey area in nursing home policies. Ask who must provide the services and under what circumstances.)

Other types of care. Adult day care provides daytime group activities in a setting outside the home. Respite care provides a secondary caregiver for an ill person while the primary caregiver gets a respite, or break, from caregiving duties.

What Is the Daily Range of Dollar Benefits?

Most long-term care policies are "indemnity" policies that offer a fixed-dollar amount each day generally ranging from $40/day to $130/day. This is the daily cash amount you will receive if you are in a nursing home. In the future, it is hoped that more policies will offer to pay a percentage of the cost. The daily payment amounts vary for different levels of care, although newer policies do not distinguish between these levels. It is important to protect yourself from inflation so consider what the dollar amount you select will be worth in 10 or 20 years.

(Presently, the average cost is between $65 to $70 per day.) Also find out if there are maximum lifetime benefits.

For How Long Will the Policy Pay Benefits in a Nursing Home?

If you are confined to a nursing home, you need to decide how long you want the policy to pay benefits. Benefits are expressed in days, units, or dollars. Some policies limit the maximum benefit, such as a limit on the number of consecutive days for which benefits will be paid. An average length of stay for patients who are admitted to a nursing home for a chronic condition and who stay there for more than 3 months is 2.5 years. Benefit options range from 2 years to lifetime coverage. A 4-year policy (1,460 days) refers to the number of days a person will collect benefits if he or she is in a nursing home. It does not refer to the length of time the person pays premiums.

Is Prior Hospitalization or Institutionalization Required Before the Policy Will Pay?

Many people who enter nursing homes for custodial care have not needed prior hospitalization or skilled care, and it is not easy for a physician to admit a person to a hospital for a few days in order to fulfill this policy requirement. Avoid policies that have this restriction, as well as those that require skilled care before paying for a lower level of care. Many states are passing legislation that prohibits these restrictions.

How Long Is the Waiting Period for Preexisting Conditions?

If your policy states that for a certain period of time from the effective date, generally 6 months, the policy will not cover you for any medical condition that you already had, and if you enter a nursing home during that waiting period, you pay for the charges.

What Is the Elimination or Deductible Period?

This refers to the number of days policyholders agree to pay their own expenses in a nursing home before benefits are paid by the company. The policyholder can choose to pay for the first 100 days, the first 20 days, or 0 days (policy takes effect immediately). The more days the policyholder is willing to pay for, the less expensive the premium.

Does the Policy Cover Alzheimer's Disease and Senile Dementias?

Look for language specifying coverage of these medical conditions. Many people enter nursing homes because of these illnesses. Alzheimer's disease and related senility *should not* be excluded.

Who Determines if Your Nursing Home Stay Is Necessary?

Will you need your own physician's certification of medical need? Or, does the company require a functional assessment by a person it hires to measure your ability to perform "activities of daily living"? Make sure you understand the company's definitions of these requirements.

Is There a Waiver of Premium?

Will the policyholder have to continue to pay the policy premiums while confined in the nursing home? Typically, after 90 days of paying daily benefits, excluding the waiting period, the premiums are waived.

What Are the Age Limits to Purchase the Policy?

Certain policies are not sold to persons over a certain age, usually 80 or 85. If they are sold to older people, benefit options are usually limited. Premiums are lower if you purchase at a younger age; however, purchasing a policy much before age 60 might mean keeping up with inflation for 30 years! Even with inflation protection, costs may rise well beyond the value of your policy's benefits.

Is the Policy Guaranteed Renewable for Life or Noncancelable?

Individual policies should be noncancelable or guaranteed renewable for life. The insured person can continue the policy in force by paying premiums on time. The insurer cannot change the terms of the policy. With guaranteed renewable policies, premiums can go up, but only for all persons in a certain class, as in one state. Unless your state regulations protect people insured by group policies, group long-term care insurance is not as secure because the insurance company and the association group, which act as the middlemen, reserve substantial rights to change premiums or benefits or to cancel the master policy or certificates altogether. Also keep in mind that should the company pay out its maximum promised benefits, it is unlikely that the buyer would be allowed to purchase additional long-term care coverage.

What Kind of Health Underwriting Is Required?

Typically, you will need a physician's report or you will need to fill out a question-and-answer form. Be truthful. Do not let an agent answer questions for you. Although most companies will not insure people with certain serious conditions, you must not withhold information because this can jeopardize future claims or cause a policy to be canceled. (A policy can only be canceled within the first 2 years, unless there is a case of fraud.)

Does the Policy Contain Nonforfeiture Benefits?

If you cancel your policy or forget to pay the premium, some policies return part of what you have paid in premiums. Usually benefits are *not* paid in cash, instead you will receive a reduced benefit. You must have paid premiums for a certain number of years before you will receive returned premiums.

What Does the Policy Cost?

Long-term care insurance can be expensive. According to the Health Insurance Association of America (HIAA), an average policy without inflation protection costs $1,135 per year for a 65-year-old person in 1989 and $3,841 for a 79-year-old person. There are, however, competitive, lower priced policies in the marketplace. Again, according to the HIAA, an average policy with inflation protection increased to $1,395 per year for a 65 year old and to $4,199 for a 79 year old. It is important to shop and compare prices and benefits. Most companies offer inflation protection for an additional cost. With this option the daily benefit selected automatically increases by a specified percentage (typically 5% of the original daily benefit) for a specified number of years. You must decide whether this increase will be adequate to keep up with rising inflation over many years. Some policies let the policyholder pay a higher rate for a period of years so that a policy can be "paid-up." After that period there can be no further premium increases.

What Would an "Ideal" Long-Term Care Policy Look Like?

An ideal long-term care policy would include the following:

1. It covers 85% of the cost of skilled, intermediate, and custodial levels of care, as well as home care, adult day care, and respite care.
2. It covers the above indefinitely.
3. No prior hospitalization or institutionalization is required to collect benefits for any of the above levels of care.
4. The policy is in full force immediately; no waiting periods for preexisting conditions.
5. It has no elimination period; it pays on first day.
6. It covers Alzheimer's disease, senile dementias, Parkinson's disease.
7. Premiums do not go up with policyholder's age.
8. It has no age limitations for initial purchase.
9. The policy is noncancelable.
10. Persons with health problems can purchase the policy even though they may have to pay a higher premium (called "guaranteed issue").
11. The company does not argue with you when it comes time to pay.
12. The premiums are low enough so that you can afford this policy.

How Can Life Insurance Cover Long-Term Care?

According to the American Council of Life Insurers, more than 50 insurers presently offer "living benefits" either as part of standard life insurance policies or as riders. These policies generally pay about 2% a month of the face value of your life insurance policy for up to 2 years in a nursing home. On a $50,000 policy, that would equal $1,000 per month. Some of these policies have an additional annual premium that may equal the cost of nursing home insurance. Of course, you first have to meet the life insurance company's qualifications. At this time no one is quite sure about the tax implications of these policies, that is, whether benefits are taxed. Proceed with caution.

What Are Some of the Living Arrangement Options in the "Continuum of Care," and Who Pays for Them?

Live in Own Home

A person living at home can hire needed services and take advantage of senior centers for recreation, adult day care, transportation services, and nutrition services such as meal sites or Meals-on-Wheels. Contact the Area Agency on Aging (AAA) in your area for available services including Meals-on-Wheels, private-case management, or transportation. All states have local federally funded AAAs, which are an excellent source of information and referrals for senior services. In some communities home- and community-based services (HCBS) may be available through the state's Medicaid program. The HCBS pays for services to those persons who are unable to care for themselves, unable to meet certain income requirements, and are in jeopardy of being placed in a nursing home.

Congregate Housing

This arrangement may provide some support services that allow an independent life-style, such as private living quarters, meals in a central dining room, transportation, social and recreational activities, housekeeping, and linen services. This is usually a private pay arrangement. Some housing may be federally subsidized, thereby reducing rent for people who qualify.

House Sharing

Several people who may be unrelated share kitchen and bath, but each person may have private space. This is a private pay arrangement.

Continuing Care Community

A continuing care community offers lifetime housing and limited access to health care services including nursing care, although there may be an increased fee for services. This is a private pay arrangement. You may have to invest your lifetime savings to qualify for entrance. You must consider what will happen if the resident is not pleased with the quality of living conditions, quality of services, or what may happen if ownership changes or the company goes bankrupt.

Assisted Living

Assisted living provides living arrangements that integrate shelter and personal services for frail elderly who are functionally and/or socially impaired. It offers residents individual assistance with activities of daily living, medication monitoring, and 24-hour protective supervision. In addition to luxury facilities, there are two other options.

- *Personal care boarding homes* may have local city or county licensing and are private pay.
- *Alternative care facilities (ACF) program* provides alternative care for low-income, frail elderly. Housing alternatives are licensed by the state and receive Medicaid dollars to care for people who would otherwise require nursing home placement.

Nursing Homes

These living arrangements provide shelter, medical, nursing, and rehabilitation services for persons requiring round-the-clock nursing supervision. Private pay (including long-term care insurance), Medicaid (if a person's income meets the state's financial eligibility), or Medicare (which only covers a small percentage of nursing home care) are methods of payment.

5

MEDICARE APPEALS

REASONS AND PROCEDURES FOR APPEALING MEDICARE DECISIONS

Why File an Appeal?

As with any system, problems can arise. With Medicare there may be problems with claims payments—denying coverage for a service or paying too little. A Medicare system of appeals offers providers and beneficiaries a grievance procedure.

Although 50% of Medicare appeals result in higher payments on behalf of the beneficiary, fewer than 3% of Medicare beneficiaries ever exercise their right of appeal. Why? It is difficult to buck this complicated system and most people need help to undertake an appeal. Even the language used to describe the different stages of appeal could dampen the most assertive consumer: *notice of noncoverage, immediate review, Utilization Review Committee,* etc. In addition, there is always the possibility of losing a hospital appeal and having to pay for your own hospital stay. It is a lot cheaper just to leave the hospital without appealing. Appeals in situations where the Medicare "approved charge" is much lower than the physician's actual charge are also discouraging because Medicare usually defends its decision by claiming that the low charge they approved is in fact the "prevailing charge" and they cannot change that fact. Despite this gloomy picture, it pays to appeal.

For Part A, the appeals process usually begins at the office of the Medicare intermediary, a Social Security office, or the Peer Review Organization (PRO). The Medicare intermediary is responsible for implementing regulations, processing claims, and determining whether services are covered. The PRO is a physician-sponsored, nongovernmental organization of health professionals. Each state has a PRO that is contracted by the federal government to make Medicare payment decisions based on medical necessity; to review hospital treatment and ambulatory surgical center care of Medicare patients before, during, and after their stay; and to determine whether care could have been provided in a less expensive setting.

For Part B, claims the process begins at the office of the Medicare carrier or a local Social Security Office.

Who Can File an Appeal?

In the case of Part A services, appeals can be initiated by hospitals, skilled nursing facilities, home health and hospice agencies, physicians, and Medicare beneficiaries. In the case of Part B services, appeals can be initiated by beneficiaries, a person acting on behalf of the beneficiary, or providers of services such as physicians. (If a physician does not accept assignment, written consent from the beneficiary must accompany the appeal request.)

What Are the Specific Circumstances in Which an Appeal to Medicare Should Be Made, and What Are the Procedures?

In order to begin an appeal, you first must have something in writing that states coverage is denied or that shows benefit payments lower than you expected. If you disagree you may take the necessary appeal steps. The written notices tell you what appeal steps you can take.

Denial of Eligibility for Medicare

Example: You apply for Social Security benefits and Medicare and learn you do not have enough work credits to be eligible.

Occasionally a person applying for Medicare is denied eligibility but will be given a reason for denial. The applicant should first apply for Medicare by filling out the standard application and requesting that it be processed. Then to appeal a denial of Medicare eligibility, submit a written appeal on the appropriate form from Social Security and include evidence proving eligibility. The appeal must be submitted within 60 days of receipt of the written notice denying eligibility. A representative from Social Security will initially review the case. If the decision is not modified, you will be informed of further appeal procedures.

Denial of Admission to a Hospital (Medicare Part A)

Example: You find out that Medicare will not pay for an inpatient hospital stay for your upcoming surgery or other treatment.

You may be told by your physician or by the hospital that Medicare will not cover the cost of an inpatient hospital stay. This might occur if the hospital staff believes the stay is not medically necessary.

How to Appeal a Denial of Admission to a Hospital

Initial denial determination. If you have been told that Medicare has denied your admission to the hospital and you wish to have the case reviewed by the PRO, you should have a written notice stating the reasons for the admission denial. The notice must contain review instructions, including the name and telephone number of the PRO.

Immediate review (Very quick first review by the PRO). You should call or write the PRO immediately, asking them to review the case. The PRO must respond within 3 working days. When the PRO looks at a case for the first time, it is called a *review.* **OR** you could request a review as follows.

Review (Quick first review by the PRO). You should call or write the PRO within 30 days asking them to review the case. The PRO has 30 days to respond.

Reconsideration (PRO's second look at case). You have 60 days to request a reconsideration in writing, by telephone, or by submitting Form SSA-2649. A request for reconsideration is filed with the Medicare intermediary, the Social Security Administration, the Railroad Retirement Board, and the PRO or the HCFA. The physician's support, in person, by telephone, or by letter, is very important in order to provide additional information to the PRO to support your case for admission.

Hearing. If the written reconsideration of the PRO is unfavorable, the PRO will notify you of further appeal rights. The next step is to request *in writing* or by filing Form HA 501.1 a hearing to be held within 60 days before a Social Security Administrative Law Judge. The amount in controversy must be more than $200. You will be notified at least 10 days in advance of the location and time of the hearing. This is an informal proceeding. You may give someone permission to represent you if you think it would be in your best interest. Of course, you may still attend even if you have selected someone to represent you. You may also have witnesses present.

Appeals council review. If you are not satisfied with the decision, the next step is to request within 60 days after the hearing decision a review by the Social Security Administration Appeals Council (located in Arlington, Virginia). This is a review of written materials. They may grant a review and issue a decision, or they may not grant a review, or they may send the case back to the Administrative Law Judge for further review. Reviews by the Appeals Council are advised only if you are planning an appeal to the Federal District Court. You may write a letter or use Form HA-520.

Court action. If the amount in question is $2,000 or more and you are not satisfied with the Appeals Council decision, you can file a civil complaint in Federal District Court. This can be done even if the Appeals Council elected not to review the case. Your request must be made within 60 days of the Appeals Council's decision. You will need to consult an attorney at this stage.

Hospital Notice of Noncoverage for a Continued Stay in the Hospital (Medicare Part A)

Example: You have been told that Medicare will not pay for your treatment if you continue to stay in the hospital, but you do not feel well enough to leave.

Hospital admissions are continually reviewed by the hospital's Utilization Review Committees and by the Peer Review Organization. If there is disagreement as to whether your continued stay in the hospital is appropriate, certain procedures must be followed. If, for example, the hospital's Utilization Review Committee feels your care is no longer necessary and/or care can be provided in a less costly setting, the hospital must seek agreement from either the PRO or your physician. If you feel you are not well enough to be discharged, then you must obtain a Notice of Noncoverage and ask for a review.

If you do not request a review after receiving the written Notice of Noncoverage and want to stay in the hospital, you will be liable for hospital costs that begin on the 3rd day after receiving the Notice of Noncoverage. Remember, though, the hospital cannot bill you for costs if it did not provide a written Notice of Noncoverage.

How to Appeal When the Hospital Tells You That Inpatient Care Is No Longer Necessary and You Disagree

First Scenario: The Hospital and Physician Agree

Notice of noncoverage. You do not feel well enough to be discharged even though your physician agrees with the hospital that you can be safely discharged. You should request a written Notice of Noncoverage from the hospital. It will state that your physician agrees with the hospital that discharge is appropriate. The notice must include appeal instructions.

Immediate review. If you are hospitalized, your liability for payment generally begins on the 3rd day after receiving the written notice if no review request is filed. However, if an "immediate review" is requested by telephone, by letter, or by filing Form SSA-2649 by noon of the 1st workday after receiving the notice, you cannot be made to pay for the hospital care until after the PRO makes its decision. The PRO must notify you by telephone and in writing within the next full workday of its review decision and your right to continue the appeal. At this point, if the PRO agrees with the physician and the hospital that your stay is not covered, the PRO issues an "initial denial determination," and the hospital can bill you beginning noon of the day after receiving the PRO's decision. **OR** you could request a review as follows.

Review. You are hospitalized and do not request a quick "immediate" review but remain in the hospital. You can ask for a PRO review at any time during your hospital stay but remember, you are liable beginning the 3rd calendar day from receiving the Notice of Noncoverage. Since the PRO has 3 working days to review this request, you could ultimately be liable for 1 or more hospital days if the review is not favorable. An unfavorable review by the PRO at this point is called an "initial denial determination."

Reconsideration. If the decision is unfavorable, you can ask for a reconsideration within 60 days of the initial denial determination no matter how much money is in controversy. In this situation, you can request a reconsideration even if an immediate review was not requested by you during your hospital stay. A request for reconsideration is filed with the Medicare intermediary, the Social Security Administration, the Railroad Retirement Board, the PRO, or the HCFA.

Hearing. If the written reconsideration is unfavorable, you can further appeal within 60 days by asking for a hearing before a Social Security Administrative Law Judge if the amount in controversy is $200 or more and if the PRO has issued a reconsideration. (You may also use Form HA 501.1.)

Appeals council review. If you are not satisfied with the hearing decision, you can request within 60 days a review by the Social Security Administration Appeals Council (located in Arlington, Virginia). This is a review of written materials. The Council may grant a review and issue a decision, or they may not grant a review, or they may send the case back to the Administrative Law Judge for further review. Reviews by the Appeals Council are advised only if you are planning an appeal to the Federal District Court. (You may also use Form HA-520 for appeal request.)

Court action. If the amount in question is $2,000 or more—for those cases that were reconsidered by the PRO—and you are not satisfied with the Appeals Council decision, you can file a civil complaint in Federal District Court. This can be done even if the Appeals Council elected not to review the case. The request must be made within 60 days of the Appeals Council's decision. You will need to consult an attorney at this stage.

Second Scenario: The Hospital and the PRO Agree but Physician Disagrees

Notice of noncoverage. If the physician disagrees with the hospital's opinion that you no longer require hospitalization, the hospital must ask the PRO to review the case before it issues a Notice of Noncoverage. If the PRO agrees with the hospital, you will receive a written Notice of Noncoverage from the hospital stating the PRO is in agreement with the hospital that your stay is no longer necessary. The notice must include appeal instructions. Also, the hospital may begin billing you for the hospital stay on the 3rd calendar day after you receive the written Notice of Noncoverage.

Immediate Review. This is actually an immediate "reconsideration" since the PRO has already seen the records. Think of this as a "Very Quick Second Look" by the PRO.

After receiving the Notice of Noncoverage, you may request by telephone or in writing, a second consideration by the PRO, called an "immediate review." Because in this case the PRO is allowed up to 3 working days from receipt of your request to complete the review, your request should be filed as soon as possible. The PRO will inform you of its decision in writing. If you are still in the hospital, you are liable for costs beginning with the 3rd calendar day after receiving the Notice of Noncoverage, even if the PRO has not yet completed its review! This means you could ultimately pay for at least 1 day of hospital care before the review is completed by the PRO.

Reconsideration. If an "immediate review" is not requested, you still have 60 days to request a reconsideration. This request can be made after being discharged from the hospital, in a case where you are liable for hospital charges. A request for reconsideration is filed with the Medicare intermediary, the Social Security Administration, the Railroad Retirement Board, the PRO, or the HCFA.

Hearing, appeals council review, court action. If the written reconsideration is unfavorable, you may within 60 days request a hearing before a Social Security Administrative Law Judge if there is $200 or more in controversy. You may also use Form HA 501.

If you need to appeal further, you may request a review by the Social Security Administration Appeals Council, or ultimately file a lawsuit in Federal District Court if $2,000 or more.

NOTE: If, while in the hospital, you miss the "immediate review" deadlines, a review can be requested within 60 days of receiving the denial notice. The PRO has 30 days to issue a reconsidered determination. Even if you do not request a review, the PRO automatically reviews the case to make sure that the hospital's determinations are correct.

Denials as Part of an "Automatic" Retrospective Review by the PRO (Medicare Part A)

Example: Months after you were in the hospital you get a letter stating that the hospital stay was not covered by Medicare.

The PRO automatically reviews a certain percentage of Medicare inpatient stays. In some cases the PRO may determine, even after you have been discharged from the hospital, that your admission or part of your hospital stay was medically unnecessary.

The PRO may notify you after you have been discharged that the hospital stay has not ben covered by Medicare. Most often you are not responsible for the charges because you could not have been expected to know the stay would not be covered (see waiver of liability).

The hospital also receives a copy of the retrospective notice if your stay should not have been covered by Medicare. The hospital, you, or the attending physician can request a reconsideration.

How to Appeal a Retrospective Review Denial by the PRO

- If coverage of a hospital stay is denied retrospectively by the PRO, a hospital, the Medicare beneficiary, or the physician can request a reconsideration.
- The appeal procedure, thereafter, is the same as described above, i.e., a hearing with an Administrative Law Judge, then an Appeals Council review and, ultimately, Federal District Court.

Denial of Skilled Nursing Facility Services (SNF), Home Health Services, and Hospice Care (Medicare Part A)

Example: You are denied a Medicare-paid admission or denied Medicare payments for a continued stay in a Medicare-approved skilled nursing facility, or you are denied services from a home health agency or a hospice agency.

Note: Beneficiaries who are told that Medicare will not approve payments for a skilled nursing facility stay should insist that the nursing home submit a claim to the Medicare intermediary requesting a coverage decision (called "demand bills"). This permits the beneficiary to continue the appeals process if necessary.

How to Appeal Denial of SNF, Home Health Care, or Hospice Care Services

Reconsideration, hearing, appeals council, court action. Initial requests for reconsideration for these services should be submitted to the Medicare fiscal intermediary or local Social Security office, *not* to the PRO. Otherwise the procedures are basically the same as for a hospital appeal. However, the amount in controversy need only be $100 or more to request a hearing by an Administrative Law Judge or a review by the Appeals Council, and only $1,000 or more for a civil suit in Federal District Court.

Denying "Outlier" Coverage (Medicare Part A)

Example: The hospital you were in wants more money for your stay than Medicare is willing to pay.

If complex medical circumstances arise when you are in the hospital that necessitate longer, more expensive treatment that the ordinary DRG payment would not cover, the hospital bills Medicare for "cost outliers" or "day outliers" (compensation in addition to the DRG payment).

The hospital, you, or the physician may ask for a reconsideration.

Denial of a Usually Covered Service (Medicare Part B)

Example: You thought Medicare was supposed to cover a particular medical service or supply and you find out they have not paid.

The Medicare carrier makes an initial determination that a service is not covered and notifies you through an Explanation of Medicare Benefits form. If you do not agree with the determination, you may first call or write the carrier to ask questions about the decision prior to beginning a formal review. This may help you decide whether to continue with an appeal.

Some reasons why usually covered services are denied include the following.

- The service was not considered "reasonable and necessary."
- There were too many visits to a provider for a service. The Medicare carrier sets up "utilizations screens" that establish an accepted number of provider visits

per month or per year. Services that exceed accepted number of visits are noted on Medicare's computers. For example, if a patient receives more than 30 inpatient visits from physicians per month or more than 30 visits in 90 days without documentation, provider visits will be "red-flagged."

- Ambulance service that was not considered necessary.
- Oxygen equipment and other durable medical equipment considered unnecessary or purchased without physician's prescription.
- More than one physician visits the patient in the hospital (called "concurrent care". For example, your family physician and a specialist visit you in the hospital on the same day. Unless Medicare has clear evidence that both services were reasonable and medically necessary, Medicare may claim that the services duplicate one another and deny the claim.
- Physical therapy reaches a "maintenance" level.
- A billing error is found.

Often there are good reasons why the above and other services were necessary, so it is advisable to appeal.

How to Appeal a Denial of a Usually Covered Service

Review. Within 6 months from the date appearing on the initial determination notice (called "Explanation of Medicare Benefits" [EOMB]), which notifies you that some or all of the services are not covered, request the Medicare carrier to review its decision. Your request may be in the form of a letter containing your name, your Medicare health insurance claim number, and the reason you disagree with the decision. You may also submit the information on Form HCFA-1964, which can be obtained from your Medicare carrier, the HCFA, or the Social Security office. This is a review of your paperwork by the carrier, but the review will be performed by someone other than the original person who issued the initial determination. Remember to attach the appropriate Explanation of Medicare Benefits form.

In order to make a strong case for your appeal, include the following information appropriate to your case.

- Letters from physicians explaining medical necessity of services
- Medical records, including operative reports ("Open record laws" permit patient access to the records, but there may be a fee.)
- Orders and prescriptions
- Medicare records (Federal law permits a beneficiary's access to Part B carrier's records; indicate to Medicare which records they should review.)

A review can take 45 days, but difficult cases may take longer. Unless a review of a specific aspect of the case is all that is needed, request a review of the entire claim. You will receive a written decision.

Carrier hearing. If you are not satisfied with the decision and if the amount in controversy is over $100, you have 6 months from the time you receive review notification to *request in writing* a carrier hearing by a hearing officer who is employed by the Medicare carrier. Revisions to the appeals process in 1988 require claimants to first go through an "on-the-record" carrier hearing in lieu of a telephone or in-person hearing. This is a paperwork review by the carrier hearing officer.

The $100 amount is reached by figuring the difference between the actual charge and the Medicare-approved charge, minus coinsurance and deductibles. Several disputed claims (claims that have been reviewed in the last 6 months) can be combined to add up to the $100 minimum.

The quickest method to request the hearing is to write a letter to the Medicare carrier (or use Form HCFA-1965). Write to the person who signed the review or to Medicare Communications. Make sure you indicate whether you will or will not appear at the hearing. Or write to the Social Security Administration's Bureau of Hearings and Appeals, but this takes longer.

The carrier notifies you of the date, place, and time of the hearing, although you do not have to appear at the hearing. Hearings can also be conducted on the telephone. The beneficiary must receive this notice at least 14 days before the hearing is scheduled. An attorney or other authorized person is permitted to represent you if you send a signed statement indicating this or if you submit Form SSA-1696.

The officer conducting the hearing should not have been involved in previous decisions on your claim. The officer must follow the HCFA regulations and will base the decision on written evidence previously submitted in addition to new evidence and statements.

Hearing before an Administrative Law Judge. Instead of a carrier hearing, if the amount in controversy is $500 or more, you have 60 days to request in writing a hearing by a Social Security Administration Administrative Law Judge. Write a letter (or use Form HA 501.1) to the carrier or to Social Security's Bureau of Hearings and Appeals at the local Part B carrier, making sure to indicate whether you will or will not appear at the hearing. You will be notified at least 10 days prior to the hearing as to its location and time. Although it may be to your advantage to do so, you do not have to attend the hearing. An attorney or other authorized person is permitted to represent you. The judge reviews the case and will send you a full explanation of the decision.

Appeals council review. If the case requires further appeal, and if the amount in controversy is $500 or more, you have 60 days to request in writing a Review of an Adverse Decision by the Social Security Appeals Council (located in Arlington, Virginia). This is a review of written materials. They may grant a review and issue a decision, or they may not grant a review, or they may send the case back to the Administrative Law Judge for further review. Reviews by the Appeals Council are advised only if you are planning an appeal to the Federal District Court. (You may use Form HA-520 to file a request.)

Court action. If the amount in question is $1,000 or more and you are not satisfied with the Appeals Council decision, you can file a civil complaint in Federal District Court. This can be done even if the Appeals Council elected not to review the case. The request must be made within 60 days of the Appeals Council's decision. You will need to consult an attorney at this stage.

Note: When a beneficiary ceases the appeals process, the decisions at that point are final, unless the Part B carrier is asked to *reopen* the case based on additional information. Usually cases must be reopened within 12 months of the decision, but there can be extensions under certain circumstances.

Getting a Lower Medicare Payment Than Expected on a Part B Claim (Medicare Part B)

Example: You are shocked to find Medicare's approved charge is 60% lower than what your physician charged.

If a processing error has caused a lower payment than expected, this can be readily adjusted without a formal review. Many low approved charges are set at the prevailing charge in your area, however, and Medicare is bound by these figures. Although it may be unlikely that a favorable result will be achieved, it sometimes pays to request a review.

Note: In the case of a nonparticipating provider, you may wish to make sure the provider has not mistakenly charged more than the amount permitted by Medicare regulations. Physicians know the maximum charge they may bill for their Medicare services. It is illegal for a nonparticipating provider to charge more. Also, remember that in cases of elective surgery, nonparticipating surgeons and assistant surgeons must inform you in writing of charges over $500. If they do not, you may not be liable for the charges.

To file an appeal, use the same procedures, as in the previous explanation for Part B appeals.

New Information Becomes Available

Example: You learn something that may affect a prior decision by Medicare.

You generally have 1 year to reopen a case when new evidence—such as a processing error that would alter a previous decision—becomes available. In cases of fraud, there is a 4-year limit. Other exceptions exist for "good cause."

Denial of "Waiver of Beneficiary Liability" (Part A or Part B)

Example: You find out that Medicare has denied certain services you thought were covered. Will you have to pay?

A "waiver of beneficiary liability" releases you from the responsibility of paying for services. It applies when you did not know and could not be expected to know (that is, you were not informed in writing) that the medical services performed were not "reasonable or necessary" or were "custodial" in nature. Or you learn that a service was not being provided under strict Medicare definition, such as the requirement that skilled nursing services be provided on an intermittent basis under the home health benefit. Under these circumstances, Medicare denies coverage.

For Part A claims. When you receive a notice that Medicare is not covering certain charges, you are usually released from liability. For example, a patient may be an inpatient in the hospital receiving rehabilitation. Upon review, the PRO discovers that the services received by the patient did not meet Medicare's time criteria. Perhaps the patient received only 2 hours of therapy per day instead of 3. The hospital will receive a copy of this notice and may be liable. In some cases the hospital does not get paid by the Medicare fiscal intermediary or may have to give money back, if it has already been paid. In cases in which the hospital did not know and could not expect to know, Medicare pays the hospital.

In some cases, the patient may be liable. For example, a patient received a Notice of Noncoverage for a previous hospitalization. If the patient then enters another hospital for the same reason the PRO assumes that the patient should have known that the stay would not be covered.

If a patient has paid a provider and has been issued a waiver of liability, Medicare will reimburse the patient if the patient requests payment in writing within 6 months after paying.

For Part B claims. A waiver of liability only applies to providers who accept assignment on the claim. Medicare notifies the provider and you that coverage is denied. You are automatically released from liability at this point, and the provider must refund any money you paid within 30 days or they must request a review. If the provider can prove that you knew the services would not be covered (you signed a statement to that effect), then you may be liable for the payment. If neither the provider nor you could have been expected to know that expenses were excluded from coverage, Medicare will pay the provider. Otherwise, the provider must absorb the loss. Medicare notifies both the provider and you of the outcome after a review.

Note: Physicians are prohibited from having patients routinely sign statements acknowledging that Medicare may not pay for the service.

If services have been supplied by a provider who did not accept Medicare assignment, you may not be liable for charges if Medicare decides the services are "not reasonable and necessary." If the provider knew or should have known that services would not be covered by Medicare, the physician must give written notice explaining why he or she believes Medicare is likely to deny payment before performing the service. The physician must also get your written agreement to pay for the services. If written notice is not given, you do not have to pay if services were denied because they were "not reasonable and necessary" (unless the physician did not know or could not reasonably have been expected to know that Medicare would not pay for the services). Any payments you made to the physician must be refunded to you within 30 days. Remember if you did not sign a statement prior to treatment but think your treatment may not be "reasonable and necessary," make sure you ask the physician to submit the claim to Medicare for you.

How to Appeal a Denial of Waiver of Liability

Review. If you are requesting the review, it is important that you submit convincing evidence that you could not have known Medicare would not cover the services in question. For Part A services, first appeal to the PRO or the Medicare intermediary. For Part B services, first appeal to the Medicare carrier.

Hearing, appeals council review, court action. If the decision is unfavorable, continue the same procedures for Part A or Part B appeals as described above.

Denial of Coverage Made by Health Maintenance Organizations (HMOs) or Competitive Medical Plans (CMPs)

Example: Your HMO or CMP does not cover something you thought was covered.

The appeal rights are similar to the rights of traditional fee-for-service Medicare beneficiaries. If you disagree with the initial decision of the HMO or CMP, follow the steps listed on the preceding pages.

The HMOs and CMPs that have contracts with Medicare are required to give each enrollee a written explanation of appeal rights.

Reminders

Keep copies of everything.

- Keep good notes—noting names of persons to whom you speak and dates. Paperwork gets lost!
- Do not wait too long to begin appeals.

Review of Appeals Procedures

Steps of Part A Appeals

1. Depending on circumstances, request within 60 days an immediate review, or a reconsideration from the PRO or intermediary.
2. Request within 60 days a hearing by a Social Security Administrative Law Judge if amount in dispute is $100 or more ($200 or more for cases reconsidered by the PRO).
3. File for a review with the Social Security Appeals Council within 60 days if amount in dispute is $100 or more ($200 or more for cases reconsidered by the PRO).
4. File civil action in Federal District Court within 60 days if amount in dispute is $1,000 or more ($2,000 or more for cases reconsidered by the PRO).

Steps of Part B Appeals

1. Request a review within 6 months, or request a reopening or adjustment—if you simply need to correct something—within a year.
2. Request a carrier hearing within 6 months if amount in dispute is over $100, or request an administrative law judge (ALJ) hearing within 60 days if amount in dispute is over $500.
3. File for a review with the Social Security Appeals Council if amount in dispute is over $500.
4. File civil action in Federal District Court if amount in dispute is over $1,000.

6

FILING CLAIMS AND ORGANIZING THE PAPERWORK

HOW TO FILE CLAIMS

Who Files Claims to Medicare?

Part A claims are almost always filed by an institution, such as a hospital, nursing home, home health agency, or hospice agency. Medicare sends any reimbursement directly to the provider.

Effective September 1, 1990, there is a mandatory claim filing requirement. All Part B claims, whether "assigned" or "unassigned" must be filed to Medicare by service providers—physicians, laboratory, medical supply company, and others. These providers are prohibited from charging patients for submitting these claims for them. If the provider accepts a Medicare assignment, Medicare pays the provider directly. If the provider does not accept assignment, payment is made to the patient. Almost all hospitals participate in Medicare and, therefore, accept assignment, so hospitals receive payment directly from Medicare for Part B outpatient services.

What Coding System Is Used by Providers When Sending Bills to Medicare?

Providers must list Medicare services, supplies, and diagnoses using the formal coding system of letters and numbers in addition to a written description. The system used is the Health Care Financing Administration Common Procedure Coding System, nicknamed HCPCS (pronounced "hick picks").

Procedure Codes

There are three levels of codes used for patient procedures.

Level 1: Physicians' Current Procedural Terminology (CPT-4). This book lists more than 7,000 physician procedures and services and is updated annually by the American Medical Association (AMA). Most insurance companies require that services be listed according to these codes, which are composed of five numbers.

90017 "New patient" has an "extended service" office visit

Level 2: National Codes. This manual supplements the CPT-4 book, listing more than 2,500 codes for supplies and services that are not contained in CPT-4 but that may be covered by Medicare and Medicaid. These codes are arranged alphanumerically; they start with a letter (A through V) and are followed by four numbers.

J0290 Injection, Ampicillin, up to 500 MG
E1280 Heavy Duty Wheelchair, detachable arms(desk or full length), elevating leg rests

Level 3: Local Codes. Each Medicare carrier can create its own codes for use in the region it administers. They must obtain government approval before using these local codes. These codes are also arranged alphanumerically; however, they begin with the letter Y, followed by four numbers (some local codes use two letters followed by three numbers).

Y0715 Implantation of anti-gastroesophageal reflux device

Diagnosis Codes

In addition to a procedure code, all claim forms submitted to Medicare must also contain the patient's diagnosis in the form of a number code. These are contained in the *International Classification of Diseases, 9th Revision—Clinical Modification (ICD-9-CM).*

785.1 Palpitations
070 Viral hepatitis
157.1 Malignant neoplasm of the body of the pancreas

Why Does One Medical Visit Sometimes Incur Two Bills?

Some outpatient medical services incur both a technical fee and a professional fee. For example, if a patient goes to a hospital for an X ray, he or she may receive two bills. The hospital charges for taking the X ray including the film, equipment, etc. This is known as the "technical component" of the charge. Reading and reporting on the X ray is done by a radiologist who is a physician and who bills separately. The radiologist's bill makes up the "professional component" of the X ray.

Can a Beneficiary File a Part B Claim to Medicare?

Beneficiaries no longer have to submit claims to Medicare. If a provider refuses to submit a claim, beneficiaries should contact their Medicare carrier. Providers are subject to penalties for noncompliance.

If a provider believes a service is not covered by Medicare, but the beneficiary insists on a formal Medicare determination, providers are encouraged to submit a claim. This also applies in cases where the beneficiary needs a formal Medicare denial for supplemental insurance purposes.

Situations in which the beneficiary may file a claim and in which the provider will not be penalized include the following.

1. Foreign claims
2. Used durable medical equipment purchased from a private source
3. Services billed directly to other third-party insurers ("indirect payment provision")
4. Medicare secondary payer (MSP) claims in which the provider does not have the essential information necessary for filing the claim (In this case the beneficiary would attach the primary insurer's payment determination notice when filing to Medicare as the secondary payer. For more information about MSP claims, see section on Medicare as a second payer, this chapter.)
5. Other unique situations as determined on a case-by-case basis by the carrier

In the exceptional case in which the beneficiary submits a claim to the Medicare office of the carrier in the state where the services were received, the following procedure should be followed:

1. Complete and sign a Patient's Request for Medicare Payment (Form HCFA-1490S; see Figure 6.1 at the end of this chapter). You can request these forms by telephoning from a Social Security office or the Medicare carrier. In cases where the provider has refused to submit a claim, you should include a signed statement outlining your attempts to get the provider to submit your claim.
2. Include itemized bills (see Figure 6.2 at the end of this chapter) that contain the following.

- Date of service
- Place where service was provided
- Name of the provider
- Code describing the services
- Code for diagnosis
- Charges
- Your name and the Medicare claim number including the letter that follows it

Often the physician will give the patient this information on Form SSA 1500. If a claim is being submitted for rental or purchase of durable medical equipment, include the physician's prescription, in addition to the above information.
IMPORTANT: Always keep a copy of each of these documents for your records.

What Are the Time Limits for Filing a Claim?

Generally claims should be filed within 1 year by providers.

What Is an Explanation of Medicare Benefits (EOMB)?

The Explanation of Medicare Benefits (EOMB) is the document that Medicare mails every beneficiary to show what has (or has not) been paid on the beneficiary's claims. The EOMB notice shows what services have been covered, when they were rendered, by whom, the provider's billed charge, how much Medicare approved, how much was credited to the $100 annual deductible, and how much Medicare paid.

Whether a claim is assigned or unassigned, paid in full or denied, the beneficiary still receives an EOMB. Many beneficiaries call these forms the "This-is-not-a-bill" form because that is what is printed across the top. Indeed, these are not bills, merely a means of letting the beneficiary know about any action taken on claims filed to Medicare. Unfortunately, no matter how hard the Health Care Financing Administration and the carriers try, these documents remain very confusing for most people and often contain unclear information from Medicare.

How Do You Read an EOMB?

There are three types of EOMB notices.

1. *Inpatient stay.* (See Figure 6.3 at the end of this chapter.) Medicare beneficiaries who have been an inpatient in a hospital or skilled nursing facility should receive a Medicare Benefit Notice. Many beneficiaries complain they do not receive these notices. Always request one following an inpatient stay if it is not mailed to you.

The EOMB form for inpatient stays includes the patient's Medicare number (also called the health insurance claim number), the service provider (hospital or nursing home), the dates of the inpatient services, the benefit days used, and the payment status. For example, in Figure 6.3, Medicare paid for all covered services except $628. No deductable was applied.

2. *Part B outpatient services from a hospital, skilled nursing facility, home health agency or physical therapy provider.* (See Figure 6.4 at the end of this chapter.) Medicare beneficiaries who have received outpatient services from a facility, such as a hospital, receive an EOMB labeled Medicare Claims Information. This form lists services such as X rays taken at the hospital, emergency room services, day surgery, physical therapy, respiratory services, etc.

The form contains the patient's name, address, Medicare number (health insurance claim number) as well as the date of first service and date of last service (if services were received on one day, then these two dates will be the same). The EOMB shows provider's name and address (hospital's name and address).

This form also includes type of service provided (laboratory tests, X rays, etc.), covered charges (what the hospital charged the patient), total covered charges, Part B blood charge deductible, coinsurance (20% of covered charges excluding laboratory charges), and amount paid by Medicare. The 20% you are expected to pay to the hospital is not necessarily 20% of the Medicare-approved charge. The Medicare-approved charge could be more. The Medicare-approved charge is determined by a financial agreement between Medicare and each hospital.

This form also tells you how much of your $100 Part B deductible has been met, how much you have paid the provider, how much you still owe the provider, and the amount of refund, if any.

Note: Almost all hospitals are participating providers and therefore accept Medicare assignment.

The following example shows how to calculate charges included on the EOMB.

Maurice went to General hospital as an outpatient. The hospital's charges were $35.90 for his blood test (although $29.63 appears as the amount covered by Medicare as limited by a fee schedule), $51.20 for his X ray, and $18.05 for respiratory services. His "covered charges" were

Step 1

lab/chemistry	$29.63
X ray	51.20
respiratory services	+18.05
Total covered charges	$98.88

Step 2

Subtract charges paid at 100%. This applies to clinical diagnostic lab tests that are reimbursed by Medicare at 100% of a Medicare fee schedule.

$98.88	total covered charges
- 29.63	Medicare covers 100% of diagnostic lab
$69.25	

Step 3

Assuming the $100 deductible has been met, multiply

$69.25
× .20
$13.85

Maurice pays 20% of the covered charges as coinsurance or $13.85. Medicare then lists the balance of Medicare-covered charges at $85.03 ($29.63 + 80% [51.20 + 18.05]).

3. *Outpatient physician services (or other suppliers).* (See Figures 6.5 and 6.6 at the end of this chapter.) The format of this EOMB is different, although it gives the same standard information as in the outpatient hospital EOMB described above. Across the top it reads "Your Explanation of Medicare Benefits." Most important, this document tells who provided the services and whether or not assignment was accepted. It may read, "assignment was taken on your claim for $35 from Dr. Fixit" (the provider's name is often abbreviated beyond recognition) or "assignment was not taken on your claim for $35."

The EOMB will also show the billed amount, how much of the billed amount was approved, and how much Medicare paid (usually 80% of that amount). It will also indicate if there was any amount deducted that can be applied to your annual deductible and what the status of your deductible is for the year.

The amount Medicare pays is periodically reduced by a small percentage due to Congress's ongoing attempt to adjust the budget deficit. Known as the Gramm–Rudman deficit reduction law, it reduces Medicare payments by 1% to 2%. On assigned claims, the patient is not responsible for the difference. Therefore, you multiply 20% by the "approved charge" to find the correct amount owed.

The following example shows how a deductible on an assigned claim is calculated.

Step 1

Physician office visit charge $30.60

Step 2

Medicare approves $22.10

Step 3

Patient Part B deductible $10.00

(Medicare decides when and how much to apply toward a person's $100 annual Part B deductible.)

Step 4

$22.10 - 10.00 = $12.10

Step 5

$12.10 × .80 = $9.68 (Medicare pays 80% of the approved charge minus any deductible.)

Step 6

$22.10	approved amount
- 9.68	Medicare paid
$12.42	patient pays

Or do you want to do this last step the long way?

$12.10 × .20 =	$2.42	patient's 20% coinsurance
	+ 10.00	patient's deductible
	$12.42	patient pays

Since assignment was accepted, patient is not responsible for the $8.50 difference between the actual charge of $30.60 and the approved charge of $22.10.

How Long Does It Take to Receive the EOMB?

It can take 6–8 weeks before Medicare sends the patient an Explanation of Medicare Benefits. A check for 80% of the Medicare-approved charge is usually enclosed with the EOMB on unassigned claims. Unfortunately, EOMBs often contain information about more than one provider and checks may incorporate payments for more than one provider. This can be very confusing. The Medicare payment should be used to reimburse the medical provider, unless the provider has already been paid.

Who Should Be Contacted if Medicare Fraud or Abuse Is Suspected?

If you suspect that a physician, supplier, hospital, or other health care provider has been billing Medicare for services not performed, or performing unnecessary services, you should call the toll-free Medicare Fraud and Abuse Hot Line at 1-800-368-5779. In Maryland call 1-800-638-3986.

If you suspect fraudulent practices regarding your Medigap or long-term care insurance, you should contact your state's Insurance Commissioner.

Under What Circumstances Does Medicare Pay as a Secondary Payer?

For the majority of persons 65 or older, Medicare is the primary payer. However, there are exceptions in which Medicare is the secondary payer. This occurs when services received are covered by accident or liability insurance, Veterans Administration, Worker's Compensation, federal black lung benefits, or no-fault insurance. Medicare will pay as a secondary payer after the other coverage meets its payment responsibility. (This includes ongoing care related to injuries or illnesses that occurred in the past.)

If a person is a Medicare recipient solely because of end-stage renal disease and is covered by employee group health insurance, Medicare is the secondary payer.

If a person over age 65 (or the spouse), entitled to Part A is working and covered by an Employer Group Health Plan (EGHP), Medicare may be the secondary insurance. Companies with over 20 employees—and small subsidiaries with under 20 workers that are part of a larger company—must offer the same health plan to older employees as they do to younger employees. Older workers can decide whether their company plan or Medicare will be the primary payer. If a person elects Medicare as primary payer, the employer is not permitted to offer coverage that supplements Medicare. The person covered by the EGHP can then decide whether to enroll in Part B of Medicare to supplement the EGHP. There is no penalty or late enrollment in Part B under these circumstances (Review "Enrollment" in Chapter 1).

To review, Medicare is the primary payer for beneficiaries who are retired, for beneficiaries covered by an EGHP with fewer than 20 employees, and for employed beneficiaries who select Medicare as a primary payer.

Will Medicare Pay if You Have an Accident?

Yes, but if you have other liability or accident insurance, Medicare pays as a secondary insurance. For certain diagnoses, Medicare requires information from the patient to find out whether an accident was involved and whether another party is liable as primary insurer. Many Medicare beneficiaries receive letters from Medicare requesting this information and are often confused by them. The beneficiary should answer the questions and return the form promptly so there is no delay in future claims processing. In cases where another liability insurer may be responsible, the claim should be filed to Medicare first. Medicare will make a conditional payment and then recover the conditional payments after the liability settlement amount is paid.

What Procedure Should Be Followed When a Beneficiary Dies?

In the event of a beneficiary's death, Part A providers send assigned claims to Medicare. Medicare will make payments directly to the Part A provider.

When Part B claims remain unpaid after the death of the beneficiary, Medicare will only forward reimbursement to a provider who accepts Medicare assignment.

If assignment is not accepted, Medicare will send a letter to a responsible party, such as a spouse. Medicare cannot make payment on a claim until someone assumes responsibility, which releases Medicare from liability. Those representing the deceased can ask the physician or provider to resubmit the claim as an "assigned claim" so that Medicare will reimburse the provider directly. Often, those representing the deceased will also give the provider permission to bill the Medicare supplemental insurance on behalf of the deceased policyholder.

If the provider will not accept Medicare assignment, the spouse or other representative can offer to sign an HCFA Form 1660 (Request for Information-Medicare Payment For Services of a Patient Now Deceased). (See Figure 6.7 at the end of this chapter.) By signing this form, the person representing the deceased agrees to be responsible for paying the physician/provider in full. The provider submits the unassigned claim. Medicare will send the checks to this representative.

What Is the Procedure for Filing Medicare Supplemental Insurance Claims?

It is a good idea to fill out and keep a sample claim form handy to simplify future claim filing. If necessary, call the insurance company to find out what information is needed. Ask where you should sign your name and whether you will receive payments directly or have them forwarded to the provider.

When filing Medicare supplemental claims you should follow the procedures below.

1. Mail the following to the company.
   - The company's insurance claim form
   - A copy of the Explanation of Medicare Benefits
   - If required, a copy of the physician's itemized bill, which includes the name of the physician, the date of the service, the services rendered including diagnosis, and the actual charge
2. Keep a record of the date documents were mailed to the insurance company with your copies of the documents. (The physician's office or other provider may also mail a claim to your supplemental insurance if you give them authority.) You will receive an Explanation of Benefits (EOB) from your insurance company that explains what has been paid on each claim.
3. Keep track of where the company mails the supplemental insurance checks (e.g., to the physician directly, or to the policyholder directly?). This part gets confusing if a person has already paid the physician and the insurance company sends its check to the physician. Keep careful records.
4. Deposit all checks from the insurance company into personal accounts and pay providers by personal check when a bill is received. It is a good idea to write the date received and amount directly on the EOB for future reference.

HOW TO ORGANIZE PAPERWORK

What Is the Best Procedure for Organizing Medical Billing Paperwork?

EXAMPLE

Mrs. Peres, a 68-year-old widow who lives alone, recently returned home after 30 days in the hospital. She had been diagnosed with lung cancer and had her left lung removed. While she was in the hospital, she developed a blood clotting disorder and had to have her left leg amputated below the knee. She was home for 2 months and needed oxygen while she was recovering. The amputation did not heal properly, however, and she had to go back in the hospital in July to have more of the leg amputated. She was fitted with a prosthesis within a month after the second surgery.

Compounding her illness were the piles of bills and statements arriving daily in the mail. She had to sort through medical bills and statements, Medicare Explanations of Benefits, and assemble paperwork to submit to her supplemental insurance. The sheer quantity of paperwork in this case was overwhelming. She began to worry about the bills, and yet she was not able to sort through the masses of paperwork and was not sure who had been paid and when.

Even though Mrs. Peres is a retired lawyer and accustomed to handling enormous amounts of paperwork, she found it very difficult to cope with the volumes of paperwork because of her physical condition. Her family, too, did not have the time nor the skill to keep up.

Many people need trained help with medical bills and statements, especially when they are recuperating from a serious illness. Some states provide trained volunteer senior health insurance counseling programs. Check with senior publications, your local Area Agency on Aging, the Division of Insurance or your local AARP chapter for information and referral. Also, there may be people who for a fee will assist you with claim filing.

If you tackle "the insurmountable pile" yourself, try to focus on one step at a time. Do not worry about trying to accomplish everything in one sitting. It may take hours. Go at your own pace. You will probably develop your own way of doing things, but here are a few hints.

1. Remove all papers from envelopes and discard the envelopes, not the bills. This often lightens the load significantly.
2. Separate papers into files by provider, such as physician, hospital, or a supplier. Each provider file should include bills, statements, Explanations of Medicare Benefits, and Explanations of Benefits from the supplemental insurance company, as well as any collection notices for the service.
3. Organize each provider file by date of service. Sometimes there is only one document indicating that a service was performed on a certain day. Search for clues carefully.
4. Start with one provider at a time and begin to fill in a record-keeping form (you may design your own form or use the sample form [Figure 6.8] at the end of this chapter).

Use pencil only. Indicate each date of service for that provider. Starting left to right on the form, fill in whatever information you already know about that service. Use one record-keeping form per provider. Put a check mark on each document to show you have entered it.

The most important document is the Explanation of Medicare Benefits. It should give accurate information about date of service, provider, whether assignment was accepted, amount billed, amount approved, amount paid by Medicare, and a record of your Part B $100 deductible. This information should be copied onto your record-keeping form. You should keep a record of amounts applied toward the annual $100 deductible.

5. When all dates of service for all providers have been entered, review the record-keeping form and decide what action, if any, to take.

   - Send any claims to Medicare
   - Send any claims to supplemental insurance
   - Call the physician's office for itemized bills
   - Call Medicare for copies of EOMBs
   - Forward any payments to the physician (only if physician or provider has sent you a statement of payments due)

If you do take any action, keep careful notes of what you did in the "comments" spaces provided. For example, if you call Medicare, write "12/4/89—called Medicare for copy of EOMB"; "10/10/89—spoke to Judy in Dr. K's office; she'll rebill Medicare"; "2/1/90—mailed Dr. C $15.12, check #1213."

If you think you should have already received an EOMB or if it is missing, write or call your Medicare office. Give the beneficiary's name, Medicare claim number, date of service, amount of the service, and name of provider. Medicare will not give information over the phone to anyone except the beneficiary or an authorized representative.

6. File a claim to the supplemental insurance when you have the following.

   - A copy of the Explanation of Medicare Benefits
   - A copy of the provider's itemized bills (if the company requires this document)
   - The supplemental insurance company's claim form

   Remember to keep track of the date claims were mailed and who mailed them on your record-keeping form. When the company mails you the Explanation of Benefits, it will include information about any payments made (or not made). Fill in this information in the appropriate box on your form so you are up to date on any communications from the company. Make sure you keep a record of your insurance plan's deductible on the record-keeping form.

7. Once the initial record-keeping file is set up, you can enter additional dates of service on the appropriate record-keeping sheet for that provider when you get new documents. Any bill from a provider, a check from Medicare or the patient's supplemental insurance, or Explanations of Benefits from Medicare or from the insurance company should prompt you to review the status of your date-of-service file.
8. Ultimately, the "balance owed by patient" column should be zero.

Some Commandments to Remember

1. Always keep a copy of *everything*. Maybe some day all beneficiaries will routinely get mailed two copies of each EOMB!
2. Always record dates, *including the year*, whenever you call or write for information. You will be amazed how fast the years go by!

3. Write directly on the EOMB and the supplemental EOB the date you receive a check, the check number and amount, and what you did with the check (cashed it, deposited to checking account, etc.).

What Kind of Record-Keeping System Should Be Used to Keep Track of Paperwork?

You may wish to develop your own record-keeping system. However, the form used by the Senior Health Insurance Counseling Program in Colorado (see Figure 6.8 at end of chapter) is designed so that all essential claim information can be reviewed at a glance. When filling out this form, use a pencil so you can make changes, if necessary.

The following describes how to use this form.

1. *Date of Service.* Enter the date the service was provided.
2. *Provider or MD.* Enter the name of the physician and include the physician's group or corporate name, or other provider, for example, EKG Services, Inc., Home Health Supplies, Inc. etc.
3. *Service.* Enter the type of service provided, such as office visit (OV), lab work, mammogram, Holter monitor, etc.
4. *Charge for Service.* Enter the amount the provider actually billed.
5. *Date Sent to Medicare.* This is an optional column; enter information only if you need to know the date when the provider filed or, in rare cases, if you filed a claim.
6. *Received From Medicare.* Enter the date that Medicare sent you the EOMB (usually found at the top section of the EOMB). This date is different from the date of service.
7. *Amount Approved.* Enter the amount approved by Medicare, as listed on the EOMB.
8. *Medicare Amount Paid.* Enter the amount Medicare paid, as listed on the EOMB. (This is usually 80% of the approved charge, sometimes minus the small percentage for deficit reduction.)
9. *Patient's Balance.* For unassigned claims you owe the provider's actual billed charge. Enter the difference between the billed charge and what Medicare approved. You owe this amount plus the amount Medicare paid you plus any deductable.

   For assigned claims, subtract the amount Medicare paid from the amount approved, and enter this amount. In this case, you only owe the patient's balance amount, plus any deductible still outstanding.

10. *Assignment Accepted Yes/No.* The EOMB tells you if the claim is assigned or unassigned. Answer yes or no; it makes calculations easier.
11. *Comments.* Your notes go here.
12. *Date Sent to Supp/by Whom.* Fill in the date the claim was mailed to the supplemental insurance. Use initials of the person who sent it.
13. *Amount/Date Received.* Fill in the amount that the supplemental policy paid and the date the EOB was sent to you. This amount may cover all of or part of the amount in the patient's balance column, depending on what kind of insurance you have.
14. *Check Pay to.* Fill in who received the check, you or the provider?
15. *Patient's Remaining Balance.* To calculate this running balance, keep subtracting any payments made to a provider. For unassigned claims, subtract any payments made to the provider by you or your insurance supplement from the charge for service (although Medicare does not pay the provider directly, the supplemental insurance company may). For assigned claims, subtract from the Medicare-approved charge any payments made to the provider, by Medicare, by the supplemental insurance company, or by your personal checks.
16. *Awaiting Bills From Provider.* Enter yes or no. It is best to pay only after you actually get a bill, not before, so payments can be properly credited.
17. *Date/Amount Patient Payment.* Enter any payments made by you. Note date, amount, and check number.
18. *Comments.* This is another work column. Keep track of any amount credited toward deductibles for each calendar year.

FORM APPROVED
OMB NO 0938-0008

PATIENT'S REQUEST FOR MEDICAL PAYMENT

IMPORTANT—SEE OTHER SIDE FOR INSTRUCTIONS

PLEASE TYPE OR PRINT INFORMATION — MEDICAL INSURANCE BENEFITS SOCIAL SECURITY ACT

NOTICE: Anyone who misrepresents or falsifies essential information requested by this form may upon conviction be subject to fine and imprisonment under Federal Law. No Part B Medicare benefits may be paid unless this form is received as required by existing law and regulations (20 CFR 422.510).

1	Name of Beneficiary from Health Insurance Card (First) (Middle) (Last)	**SEND COMPLETED FORM TO:**
2	Claim Number from Health Insurance Card	Patient's Sex ☐ Male ☐ Female
3	Patient's Mailing Address (City, State, Zip Code) Check here if this is a new address ☐ (Street or P.O. Box — Include Apartment Number) (City) (State) (Zip)	3b Telephone Number (Include Area Code) ( )
4	Describe the Illness or Injury for which Patient Received Treatment	4b Was condition related to: A. Patient's employment ☐ Yes ☐ No B. Accident ☐ Auto ☐ Other 4c Was patient being treated with chronic dialysis or kidney transplant? ☐ Yes ☐ No

5

a. Are you employed and covered under an employee health plan? ☐ Yes ☐ No

b. Is your spouse employed and are you covered under your spouse's employee health plan? ☐ Yes ☐ No

c. If you have any medical coverage other than Medicare, such as private insurance, employment related insurance, State Agency (Medicaid), or the VA, complete:
Name and Address of other insurance, State Agency (Medicaid), or VA office

Policy or Medical Assistance No.

Policyholders Name:

NOTE: If you DO NOT want payment information on this claim released, put an (X) here ☐

I AUTHORIZE ANY HOLDER OF MEDICAL OR OTHER INFORMATION ABOUT ME TO RELEASE TO THE SOCIAL SECURITY ADMINISTRATION AND HEALTH CARE FINANCING ADMINISTRATION OR ITS INTERMEDIARIES OR CARRIERS ANY INFORMATION NEEDED FOR THIS OR A RELATED MEDICARE CLAIM. I PERMIT A COPY OF THIS AUTHORIZATION TO BE USED IN PLACE OF THE ORIGINAL, AND REQUEST PAYMENT OF MEDICAL INSURANCE BENEFITS TO ME.

6	Signature of Patient (If patient is unable to sign, see Block 6 on reverse)	6b Date signed

IMPORTANT
ATTACH ITEMIZED BILLS FROM YOUR DOCTOR(S) OR SUPPLIER(S) TO THE BACK OF THIS FORM

FORM HCFA-1490S (7-85) — DEPARTMENT OF HEALTH AND HUMAN SERVICES—HEALTH CARE FINANCING ADMINISTRATION

Figure 6.1 Patient's Request for Medicare Payment

HOW TO FILL OUT THIS MEDICARE FORM

Medicare will pay you directly when you complete this form and attach an itemized bill from your doctor or supplier. Your bill does not have to be paid before you submit this claim for payment, but you MUST attach an itemized bill in order for Medicare to process this claim.

FOLLOW THESE INSTRUCTIONS CAREFULLY:

A. Completion of this form.

Block 1. Print your name **exactly** as it is shown on your Medicare Card.

Block 2. Print your Health Insurance Claim Number including the letter at the end **exactly** as it is shown on your Medicare card. Check the appropriate box for the patient's sex.

Block 3. Furnish your mailing address and include your telephone number in Block 3b.

Block 4. Describe the illness or injury for which you received treatment. Check the appropriate box in Blocks 4b and 4c.

Block 5a. Complete this Block if you are between the ages of 65 and 69 and enrolled in a health insurance plan where you are currently working.

Block 5b. Complete this Block if you are between the ages of 65 and 69 and enrolled in a health insurance plan where your spouse is currently working.

Block 5c. Complete this Block if you have any medical coverage other than Medicare. Be sure to provide the Policy or Medical Assistance Number. You may check the box provided if you do not wish payment information from this claim released to your other insurer.

Block 6. Be sure to sign your name. If you cannot write your name, make an (X) mark. Then have a witness sign his or her name and address in Block 6 too.

If you are completing this form for another Medicare patient you should write (By) and sign your name and address in Block 6. You also should show your relationship to the patient and briefly explain why the patient cannot sign.

Block 6b. Print the date you completed this form.

B. Each itemized bill MUST show all of the following information:

- Date of each service
- Place of each service
  - —Doctor's Office
  - —Outpatient Hospital
  - —Patient's Home
  - —Independent Laboratory
  - —Nursing Home
  - —Inpatient Hospital
- Description of each surgical or medical service or supply furnished.
- Charge for EACH service.
- Doctor's or supplier's name and address. Many times a bill will show the names of several doctors or suppliers. IT IS VERY IMPORTANT THE ONE WHO TREATED YOU BE IDENTIFIED. Simply circle his/her name on the bill.
- It is helpful if the diagnosis is shown on the physician's bill. If not, be sure you have completed Block 4 of this form.
- Mark out any services on the bill(s) you are attaching for which you have already filed a Medicare claim.
- If the patient is deceased please contact your Social Security office for instructions on how to file a claim.
- Attach an Explanation of Medicare Benefits notice from the other insurer if you are also requesting Medicare payment.

COLLECTION AND USE OF MEDICARE INFORMATION

We are authorized by the Health Care Financing Administration to ask you for information needed in the administration of the Medicare program. Authority to collect information is in section 205 (a), 1872 and 1875 of the Social Security Act, as amended.

The information we obtain to complete your Medicare claim is used to identify you and to determine your eligibility. It is also used to decide if the services and supplies you received are covered by Medicare and to insure that proper payment is made.

The information may also be given to other providers of services, carriers, intermediaries, medical review boards, and other organizations as necessary to administer the Medicare program. For example, it may be necessary to disclose information about the Medicare benefits you have used to a hospital or doctor.

With one exception, which is discussed below, there are no penalties under social security law for refusing to supply information. However, failure to furnish information regarding the medical services rendered or the amount charged would prevent payment of the claim. Failure to furnish any other information, such as name or claim number, would delay payment of the claim.

It is mandatory that you tell us if you are being treated for a work related injury so we can determine whether worker's compensation will pay for the treatment. Section 1877 (a) (3) of the Social Security Act provides criminal penalties for withholding this information.

☆U.S. Government Printing Office: 1986—608-697

Figure 6.1 Continued

Harrison Parks
989 Spring Drive
Pueblo, CO 80011

HEALTH INSURANCE CLAIM FORM
(CHECK APPLICABLE PROGRAM BLOCK BELOW)
FORM APPROVED OMB NO 0938-0008

[X] MEDICARE (MEDICARE NO) [ ] MEDICAID (MEDICAID NO) [ ] CHAMPUS (SPONSOR'S SSN) [ ] CHAMPVA (VA FILE NO) [ ] FECA BLACK LUNG (SSN) [ ] OTHER (CERTIFICATE SSN)

PATIENT AND INSURED (SUBSCRIBER) INFORMATION

1. PATIENT'S NAME (LAST NAME, FIRST NAME, MIDDLE INITIAL): Parks, Harrison A.
2. PATIENT'S DATE OF BIRTH: 09 | 05 | 06
3. INSURED'S NAME (LAST NAME, FIRST NAME, MIDDLE INITIAL): Parks, Harrison A.
4. PATIENT'S ADDRESS (STREET, CITY, STATE, ZIP CODE): 989 Spring Drive, Pueblo, CO 80011, 714-232-0989
5. PATIENT'S SEX: MALE [X] FEMALE [ ]
6. INSURED'S ID NO (FOR PROGRAM CHECKED ABOVE, INCLUDE ALL LETTERS): 666-00-7777A
7. PATIENT'S RELATIONSHIP TO INSURED: SELF [X] SPOUSE [ ] CHILD [ ] OTHER [ ]
8. INSURED'S GROUP NO (OR GROUP NAME OR FECA CLAIM NO): Retired
[ ] INSURED IS EMPLOYED AND COVERED BY EMPLOYER HEALTH PLAN
9. OTHER HEALTH INSURANCE COVERAGE (ENTER NAME OF POLICYHOLDER AND PLAN NAME AND ADDRESS AND POLICY OR MEDICAL ASSISTANCE NUMBER): American Life & Casualty
10. WAS CONDITION RELATED TO
A. PATIENT'S EMPLOYMENT: YES [ ] NO [X]
B. ACCIDENT: AUTO [ ] OTHER [X]
11. INSURED'S ADDRESS (STREET, CITY, STATE, ZIP CODE): 989 Spring Drive, Pueblo, CO 80011
TELEPHONE NO. 714-232-0989
11a. CHAMPUS SPONSOR'S STATUS: [ ] ACTIVE DUTY [ ] DECEASED [ ] RETIRED; BRANCH OF SERVICE
12. PATIENT'S OR AUTHORIZED PERSON'S SIGNATURE (READ BACK BEFORE SIGNING)
I AUTHORIZE THE RELEASE OF ANY MEDICAL INFORMATION NECESSARY TO PROCESS THIS CLAIM. I ALSO REQUEST PAYMENT OF GOVERNMENT BENEFITS EITHER TO MYSELF OR TO THE PARTY WHO ACCEPTS ASSIGNMENT BELOW
SIGNED Signature on File DATE
13. I AUTHORIZE PAYMENT OF MEDICAL BENEFITS TO UNDERSIGNED PHYSICIAN OR SUPPLIER FOR SERVICE DESCRIBED BELOW
Signature on File
SIGNED (INSURED OR AUTHORIZED PERSON)

PHYSICIAN OR SUPPLIER INFORMATION

14. DATE OF: 03/19/90 ILLNESS (FIRST SYMPTOM) OR INJURY (ACCIDENT) OR PREGNANCY (LMP)
15. DATE FIRST CONSULTED YOU FOR THIS CONDITION: 03/19/90
16. IF PATIENT HAS HAD SAME OR SIMILAR ILLNESS OR INJURY, GIVE DATES
16a. IF EMERGENCY CHECK HERE [X]
17. DATE PATIENT ABLE TO RETURN TO WORK
18. DATES OF TOTAL DISABILITY FROM THROUGH
DATES OF PARTIAL DISABILITY FROM THROUGH
19. NAME OF REFERRING PHYSICIAN OR OTHER SOURCE (e.g., PUBLIC HEALTH AGENCY)
20. FOR SERVICES RELATED TO HOSPITALIZATION GIVE HOSPITALIZATION DATES: ADMITTED DISCHARGED
21. NAME & ADDRESS OF FACILITY WHERE SERVICES RENDERED (IF OTHER THAN HOME OR OFFICE): County Community Hospital Pueblo, CO 80011
22. WAS LABORATORY WORK PERFORMED OUTSIDE YOUR OFFICE? YES [ ] [ ] NO CHARGES
23. DIAGNOSIS OR NATURE OF ILLNESS OR INJURY. RELATE DIAGNOSIS TO PROCEDURE IN COLUMN D BY REFERENCE NUMBERS 1, 2, 3, ETC. OR DX CODE
1. 789.0 Pain, Abdominal, Acute
2. 574.0 Cholelithiasis
3.
4.

B. EPSDT YES [ ] [ ] NO; FAMILY PLANNING YES [ ] [ ] NO
PRIOR AUTHORIZATION NO.

24.

A DATE OF SERVICE FROM	TO	B* PLACE OF SERVICE	C PROCEDURE CODE (IDENTIFY)	FULLY DESCRIBE PROCEDURES, MEDICAL SERVICES OR SUPPLIES FURNISHED FOR EACH DATE GIVEN (EXPLAIN UNUSUAL SERVICES OR CIRCUMSTANCES)	D DIAGNOSIS CODE	E CHARGES	F DAYS OR UNITS	G* T.O.S.	H LEAVE BLANK
03/19/90		2	90529	Emergency Services, Comprehensive	1,2	210 00	1	1	
03/19/90		2		Admitted to Hospital	1,2		1	1	

25. SIGNATURE OF PHYSICIAN OR SUPPLIER (INCLUDING DEGREE(S) OR CREDENTIALS) (I CERTIFY THAT THE STATEMENTS ON THE REVERSE APPLY TO THIS BILL AND ARE MADE A PART THEREOF)
Richard Specks, M.D.
Co Lic # 088088
05/03/90
26. ACCEPT ASSIGNMENT (GOVERNMENT CLAIMS ONLY) (SEE BACK): YES [X] [ ] NO
27. TOTAL CHARGE: 210 00
28. AMOUNT PAID: 184 47
29. BALANCE DUE: 25.53
30. YOUR SOCIAL SECURITY NO.: 666-00-7777
31. PHYSICIAN'S SUPPLIER'S AND OR GROUP NAME, ADDRESS, ZIP CODE AND TELEPHONE NO.
Emergency Room Physicians'Billing
P.O. Box5467
Oklahoma City, OK 73143
ID NO. 84-234123
32. YOUR PATIENT'S ACCOUNT NO.: 34567-90
33. YOUR EMPLOYER ID NO.: 43341

*PLACE OF SERVICE AND TYPE OF SERVICE (T.O.S.) CODES ON BACK
REMARKS
APPROVED BY AMA COUNCIL ON MEDICAL SERVICE 6/83
FORM HCFA-1500 (1-84) FORM OWCP-1500 FORM CHAMPUS-501 (1-84) FORM RRB-1500 AMA OP-503
790-0029 (AMA OP-503) 2-PLY

Figure 6.2 Itemized Bill

U.S. DEPARTMENT OF HEALTH AND HUMAN SERVICES/HEALTH CARE FINANCING ADMINISTRATION

MEDICARE BENEFIT NOTICE

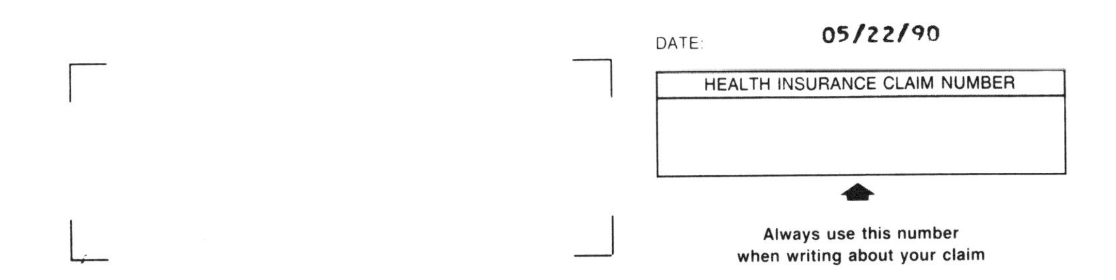
DATE: 05/22/90

HEALTH INSURANCE CLAIM NUMBER

Always use this number when writing about your claim

This notice shows what benefits were used by you and the covered services not paid by Medicare for the period shown in item 1. See other side of this form for additional information which may apply to your claim.

1 SERVICES FURNISHED BY	DATE(S)	BENEFITS USED
PRESBYTERIAN AURORA PATIENT FINANCIAL SERVICE AURORA CO 80256	04/13/90 THRU 04/27/90	14 INPATIENT HOSPITAL DAYS

2 PAYMENT STATUS

MEDICARE PAID ALL COVERED SERVICES.

IF AUTOMOBILE OR LIABILITY INSURANCE, WORKERS' COMPENSATION OR, IN SOME CASES, A HEALTH PLAN FOR EMPLOYEES ALSO PAYS FOR THESE SERVICES, A REFUND MAY BE DUE THE MEDICARE PROGRAM. PLEASE CONTACT US IF YOU HAVE HEALTH INSURANCE COVERAGE FROM ONE OF THESE SOURCES. IF YOU DO NOT HAVE HEALTH INSURANCE COVERAGE FROM ONE OF THESE SOURCES, YOU NEED NOT CONTACT US.

If you have any questions about this record, call or write

MEDICARE PART-A DIVISION
COLORADO FISCAL INTERMEDIARY
P.O. BOX 173480
DENVER, CO 80217
TELEPHONE NUMBER 1-303-831-3150

FORM HCFA-1533 (9-83)

☆U.S. GOVERNMENT PRINTING OFFICE: 1989–234-749

Figure 6.3 Medicare Benefit Notice

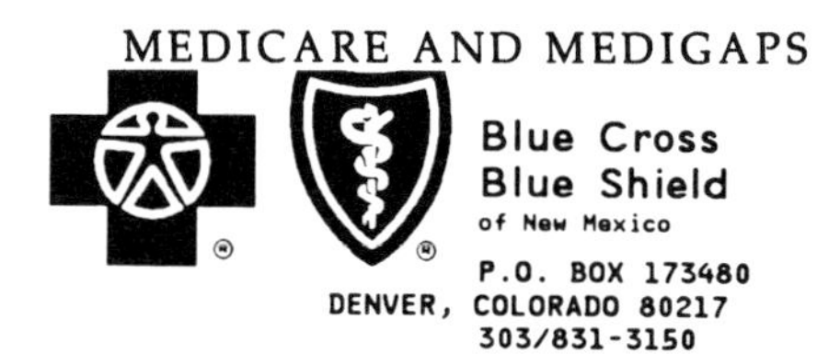

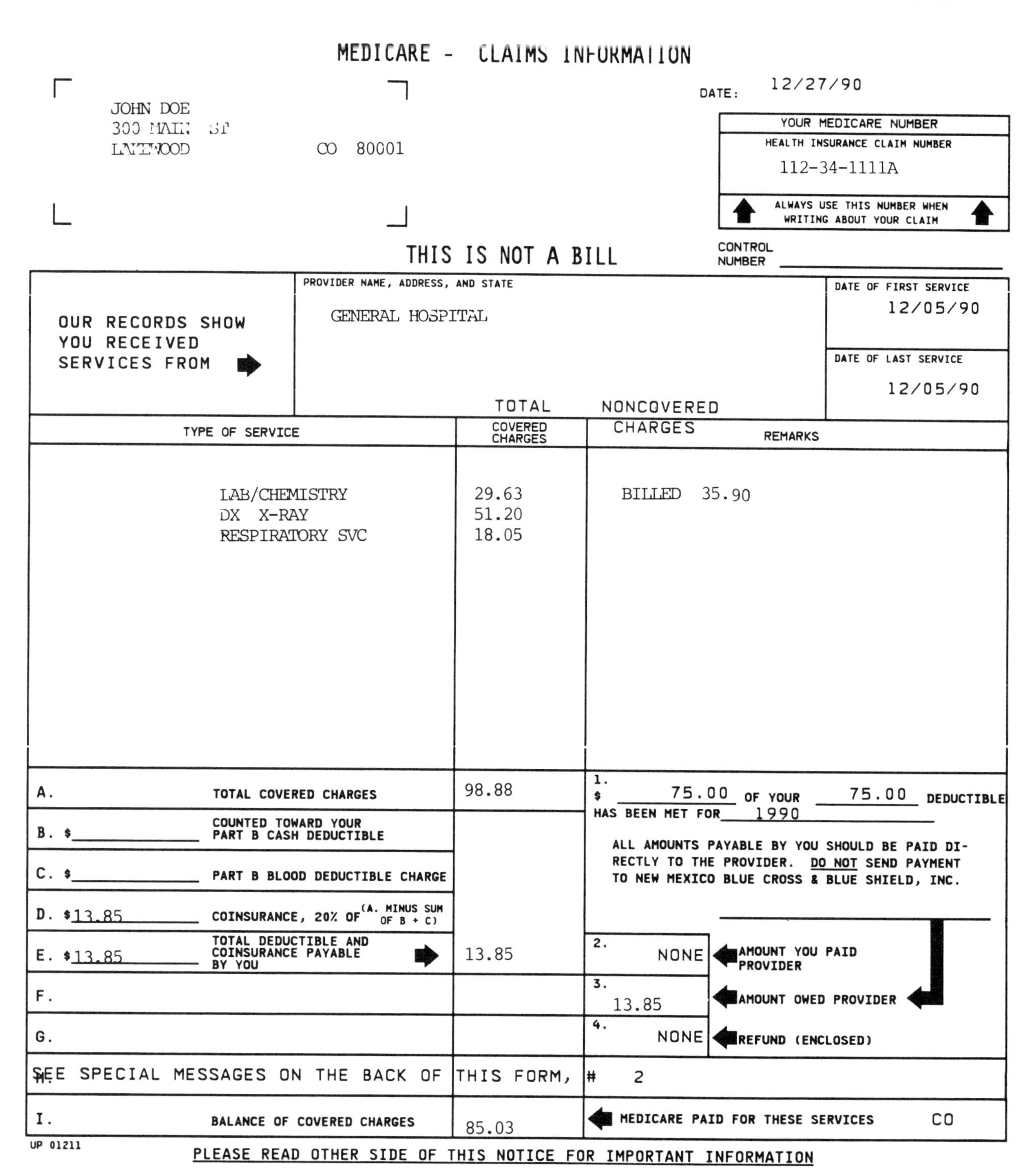

YOUR RECORD OF PART B MEDICARE BENEFITS USED
IN A HOSPITAL-SKILLED NURSING FACILITY-HOME HEALTH AGENCY-OR PHYSICAL THERAPY PROVIDER

P.O. BOX 173480
DENVER, COLORADO 80217
303/831-3150

MEDICARE - CLAIMS INFORMATION

DATE: 12/27/90

JOHN DOE
300 MAIN ST
LAKEWOOD CO 80001

YOUR MEDICARE NUMBER
HEALTH INSURANCE CLAIM NUMBER
112-34-1111A
ALWAYS USE THIS NUMBER WHEN WRITING ABOUT YOUR CLAIM

THIS IS NOT A BILL

CONTROL NUMBER

OUR RECORDS SHOW YOU RECEIVED SERVICES FROM

PROVIDER NAME, ADDRESS, AND STATE: GENERAL HOSPITAL

DATE OF FIRST SERVICE: 12/05/90
DATE OF LAST SERVICE: 12/05/90

TYPE OF SERVICE	TOTAL COVERED CHARGES	NONCOVERED CHARGES	REMARKS
LAB/CHEMISTRY	29.63	BILLED 35.90	
DX X-RAY	51.20		
RESPIRATORY SVC	18.05		

A. TOTAL COVERED CHARGES	98.88	1. $ 75.00 OF YOUR 75.00 DEDUCTIBLE HAS BEEN MET FOR 1990
B. $____ COUNTED TOWARD YOUR PART B CASH DEDUCTIBLE		ALL AMOUNTS PAYABLE BY YOU SHOULD BE PAID DIRECTLY TO THE PROVIDER. DO NOT SEND PAYMENT TO NEW MEXICO BLUE CROSS & BLUE SHIELD, INC.
C. $____ PART B BLOOD DEDUCTIBLE CHARGE		
D. $13.85 COINSURANCE, 20% OF (A. MINUS SUM OF B + C)		
E. $13.85 TOTAL DEDUCTIBLE AND COINSURANCE PAYABLE BY YOU	13.85	2. NONE AMOUNT YOU PAID PROVIDER
F.		3. 13.85 AMOUNT OWED PROVIDER
G.		4. NONE REFUND (ENCLOSED)
H. SEE SPECIAL MESSAGES ON THE BACK OF THIS FORM, # 2		
I. BALANCE OF COVERED CHARGES	85.03	MEDICARE PAID FOR THESE SERVICES CO

UP 01211

PLEASE READ OTHER SIDE OF THIS NOTICE FOR IMPORTANT INFORMATION

Figure 6.4 Explanation of Medicare Benefits (Outpatient)

YOUR EXPLANATION OF MEDICARE BENEFITS

READ THIS NOTICE CAREFULLY AND KEEP IT FOR YOUR RECORDS - THIS IS NOT A BILL

DATE OF NOTICE
OCTOBER 1, 1990

HEALTH CARE FINANCING ADMINISTRATION

MARY E KATEY
100 BROADWAY #7
DENVER, CO 80204

NEED HELP? CONTACT:
CONTRACTOR FOR
MEDICARE
Blue Cross and Blue Shield of Colorado
700 Broadway
Denver, Colorado 80273
303-831-2661
Toll Free: 1-800-332-6681
(For those living in Colorado but outside Denver Metro Area)

ASSIGNMENT WAS TAKEN ON YOUR CLAIM (CONTROL NO. 0001234567100) FOR
$ 30.60 FROM P. R. GOODWIN SEE ITEM 4 ON BACK.

		BILLED	APPROVED
1 OFFICE SERVICE(S)	AUG 1, 1990	$ 30.60	$ 22.10
APPROVED AMOUNT LIMITED BY ITEM 5C ON BACK.			

TOTAL APPROVED AMOUNT	$ 22.10
MINUS YOUR DEDUCTIBLE REMAINING FOR THIS YEAR	$ 10.00
AMOUNT REMAINING AFTER SUBTRACTING DEDUCTIBLE AMOUNT	$ 12.10
MEDICARE PAYMENT (80% OF THE APPROVED AMOUNT REMAINING)	$ 9.68

WE ARE PAYING A TOTAL OF $ 9.68 TO THOSE WHO PROVIDED THE ABOVE SERVICES. THEY AGREED TO CHARGE NO MORE FOR THE APPROVED SERVICES THAN THE AMOUNT APPROVED BY MEDICARE. YOU ARE RESPONSIBLE FOR 20 PERCENT OF THE APPROVED AMOUNT.
IF YOU HAVE OTHER INSURANCE, IT MAY HELP WITH THE PART MEDICARE DID NOT PAY.

(YOU HAVE MET THE DEDUCTIBLE FOR 1990)

IMPORTANT: If you do not agree with the amounts approved you may ask for a review. To do this you must write

to us before APR 1, 1991 (See item 1 on the back)

DO YOU HAVE A QUESTION ABOUT THIS NOTICE? If you believe Medicare paid for a service you did not receive, or there is an error, contact us immediately. Always give us the:

MEDICARE CLAIM NO.: 111223333D CLAIM CONTROL NO.: 0001234567100

FORM NO. 94642(REV. 1-90)

Figure 6.5 Explanation of Medicare Benefits (Assigned Claim)

CHECK NUMBER - 3322111 H
CHECK DATE - 09/09/90

YOUR EXPLANATION OF MEDICARE BENEFITS

READ THIS NOTICE CAREFULLY AND KEEP IT FOR YOUR RECORDS - THIS IS NOT A BILL

DATE OF NOTICE
SEP 09, 1990

HEALTH CARE FINANCING ADMINISTRATION

JOHN J HEALED

20 CHERRY LANE
AURORA CO 80111

NEED HELP? CONTACT:
CONTRACTOR FOR
MEDICARE
Blue Cross and Blue Shield of Colorado
700 Broadway
Denver, Colorado 80273
303-831-2661
Toll Free: 1-800-332-6681
(For those living in Colorado but outside Denver Metro Area)

PARTICIPATING DOCTORS AND SUPPLIERS ALWAYS ACCEPT ASSIGNMENT OF MEDICARE CLAIMS. SEE BACK OF THIS NOTICE FOR AN EXPLANATION OF ASSIGNMENT. WRITE OR CALL US FOR THE NAME OF A PARTICIPATING DOCTOR OR SUPPLIER, OR FOR A FREE LIST OF PARTICIPATING DOCTORS AND SUPPLIERS. YOUR DOCTOR OR SUPPLIER DID NOT ACCEPT ASSIGNMENT OF YOUR CLAIM (CONTROL NO. 0008765432100) TOTALING ($133.12). SEE ITEM 4 ON BACK.

		BILLED	APPROVED
A.H. KUTT :			
4 INPATIENT VISIT(S)	JULY 23-JULY 26, 1990	$ 133.12.	$ 88.00
APPROVED AMOUNT LIMITED BY ITEM 5C ON BACK.			

TOTAL APPROVED AMOUNT	$ 88.00
MEDICARE PAYMENT (80% OF THE APPROVED AMOUNT)	$ 70.40

WE ARE PAYING A TOTAL OF $ 70.40 TO YOU ON THE ENCLOSED CHECK. PLEASE CASH IT AS SOON AS POSSIBLE.
IF YOU HAVE OTHER INSURANCE, IT MAY HELP WITH THE PART MEDICARE DID NOT PAY.

(YOU HAVE MET YOUR DEDUCTIBLE FOR 1990)

IMPORTANT: If you do not agree with the amounts approved you may ask for a review. To do this you must write to us before MAR 09, 1991 (See item 1 on the back)

DO YOU HAVE A QUESTION ABOUT THIS NOTICE? If you believe Medicare paid for a service you did not receive, or there is an error, contact us immediately. Always give us the:

MEDICARE CLAIM NO.: 123456789A CLAIM CONTROL NO.:0008765432100

FORM NO. 94642(REV. 1-90)

Figure 6.6 Explanation of Medicare Benefits (Unassigned Claim)

ADDRESS INFORMATION
Mail claims to:
Beneficiary Claims
(Your local carrier's address appears here)

If you need to write to us, please use the following addresses:

- Correspondence about Medicare as secondary payor on your claims should be sent to:
(Local address of carrier appears here)
- A request for a review or other correspondence should be sent to:
(Local address of carrier appears here)

1. **DO YOU HAVE QUESTIONS ABOUT THIS CLAIM?**
If you do, call write, or visit us at the number or address shown on the other side. Call toll-free if you are outside the local area. We will tell you the facts we used to decide what and how much to approve.

If you want this claim reviewed, we will tell you how to do it. And we'll suggest other facts and proofs that you may send us. See Item 2 for your appeal rights.

If you have other questions about Medicare, read "Your Medicare Handbook." If you do not have a copy, ask a Social Security Office for one.

2. **DO YOU WANT A REVIEW OF THIS CLAIM?**
If you do not agree with the decision on this claim, you may ask to have it reviewed. The people who do the review will not be the ones who made the first decision about what and how much to approve. You may have someone help you or you can ask us for help in getting the review. Our phone number and address are shown on the other side. If the treatment was necessary in your case and the Amount Approved is less than you expected, it may help to ask your doctor for a note explaining what was done and why.

You must ask for a review in writing. You must do this not later than six months from the date of this notice, unless you have a good reason, like illness, for being late. Send you request for review to the address shown on the other side.

3. **HOW MUCH DOES MEDICARE PAY?**
You must take care of the first part of your medical bills each year. This yearly share is called the DEDUCTIBLE. After you meet the deductible, we usually pay 80% of the Amount Approved for your remaining bills. See "Your Medicare Handbook" for services that we pay at other rates.

4. **WHAT IS ASSIGNMENT?**
Assignment means your doctor or supplier of medical services agrees to accept the Amount Approved as the full amount he expects to be paid. (Participating doctors and suppliers **always** accept assignment.) With assignment, after you meet the deductible, we pay 80% and you pay 20% of the Amount Approved for most of your remaining bills. We send the check to your doctor or supplier.

5. **WHY MAY THE AMOUNT APPROVED BE LESS THAN THE AMOUNT BILLED?**
The Amount Approved is shown on the other side. It is not always the same as the current actual charge in you area. It is the lowest of the three amounts.

   a. The first is what you were charged for the service. (This is shown under "**Billed**", on the other side.)

   b. The second is the midpoint of all the charges your doctor or supplier of medical services made during a previous 12 month period for the same service. This is the **customary** charge.

   c. The third is the **prevailing** charge for your area. This is the amount which is high enough to cover the customary charge in three out of four bills for this service. This charge limit can Increase each year only by a percent set by the Government to reflect overall changes in the economy.

   If you think the payment on this claim is wrong see items 1 and 2.

6. **HOW CAN YOU USE THIS NOTICE?**
You can use it to show your doctor or others how much of your deductible you have met.

You can also send a copy to another insurance company if they need to see how much Medicare paid. They will keep the copy, so you may want to make one for yourself.

7. **WHAT ARE THE TIME LIMITS FOR FILING A REQUEST FOR MEDICARE PAYMENTS?**

These are the limits on the time you have to claim payments.

For Services Received	Send Claims By
10/1/87-9/30/88	12/31/89
10/1/88-9/30/89	12/31/90
10/1/89-9/30/90	12/31/91

You may have more time if we, the Social Security Administration, or the Health Care Financing Administration made a mistake which caused you to be late. If this happens, you must send in your claim not later than 6 months after the month the mistake was corrected.

Figure 6.6 Continued

DEPARTMENT OF HEALTH AND HUMAN SERVICES
HEALTH CARE FINANCING ADMINISTRATION

Form Approved
OMB No. 0938-0020

REQUEST FOR INFORMATION — MEDICARE PAYMENT FOR SERVICES TO A PATIENT NOW DECEASED

No further monies or other benefits may be paid out under this program unless this report is completed and filed as required by existing law and regulations (20 C.F.R. 405 1683).

When completed, send this form to:	Deceased patient
	Health insurance claim number of deceased patient

For Services Provided By:

PART I — PAID BILL (If The Bill Is Not Paid Go To Part II)

If bills for medical or other health services were paid by or for the deceased person, Medicare benefits may be due. We hope you will be able to help us determine who should receive payment. The person who paid the deceased's bill(s) has first right to any payment due. If the deceased or his estate paid the bill(s), benefits will be paid to the legal representative of the estate. If there is no legal representative, payment will be made to the person who stands highest in the list of relatives below. If the person who paid the bill(s) dies before being reimbursed, payment is also made to the person standing highest in the list of relatives. If there are no living relatives or legal representatives, no payment will be made. Please answer the questions, sign on the reverse side and return this form in the enclosed envelope.

ALWAYS INCLUDE EVIDENCE OF PAYMENT SUCH AS A RECEIPTED BILL OR OTHER RECEIPT

1. Who paid the deceased's bills for medical or other health services?

☐ The deceased or his estate *(Answer (2) below)*

☐ Yourself *(Sign on reverse side and return form)*

☐ Other person or organization (Enter the person's or organization's name and address in item 4 below. If there is more than one person or organization, attach a listing of names and addresses of these persons or organizations to this form.

2. Is there a legal representative of the estate?

☐ Yes *(If "Yes," print his name and address below, Sign on reverse side and return form).* If you are the legal representative, submit a copy of your appointment papers with this form.

☐ No *(If "No," answer item 3 below.*

3. This item is answered only if item 2 above is checked "No". Put a check in the box next to the living relative that stands highest on the following list and then write that relative's name and address in item 4 below. (If you check the box for child or children and there is more than one child, attach a listing of the names and address of all the children to this form.)

☐ Widow or widower living in the same household as the deceased at the time of death, or entitled to a monthly Social Security or Railroad Retirement benefit on the same earnings record as the deceased in the month of death.

☐ A child or children of the deceased entitled to monthly Social Security or Railroad Retirement benefits or the same earnings record as the deceased in the month of death. *(List the names and addresses of all entitled children of the deceased)*

☐ A parent or parents of the deceased entitled to monthly Social Security or Railroad Retirement benefits on the same earnings record as the deceased in the month of death.

☐ A widow or widower who was neither living with the deceased at the time of death nor at that time entitled on the same earnings record to a Social Security or Railroad Retirement benefit.

☐ A child or children of the deceased who were not entitled in the month of death to monthly Social Security or Railroad Retirement benefits on the same earnings record as the deceased. *(List the names and addresses of all such children.)*

☐ A parent or parents not entitled in the month of death to monthly Social Security or Railroad Retirement benefits on the same earnings record as the deceased.

4. Name	Address

FORM HCFA-1660 (8-81) DESTROY PRIOR EDITIONS

Continued On Back

Figure 6.7 Request for Information — Medicare Payment for Services of a Patient Now Deceased

PART II — UNPAID BILL (If The Bill Is Paid, Complete Part I)

When the beneficiary has died and a physician or supplier does not agree to accept the reasonable charge as the full charge, payment may be made on the basis of an unpaid bill to the person who has agreed to assume legal liability to pay the physician or supplier.

If you are assuming such legal liability and want to claim Medicare benefits for the services furnished to the deceased beneficiary, you must furnish the documents listed below to us and sign this form below. Your signature below certifies to the following statement:

I have assumed the legal obligation to pay the physician or supplier named below for services furnished to the deceased beneficiary on the date(s) indicated. I hereby claim any Medicare benefits due for these services.

Name of Physician or Supplier	Name of Deceased Beneficiary	Date(s) of Services

In addition furnish the following documents together with this form to us.

1. A completed form HCFA-1490S, PATIENT'S REQUEST FOR MEDICARE PAYMENTS. You must sign item 6 of the HCFA-1490S in lieu of the deceased beneficiary. (You may obtain a copy of the HCFA-1490S from a Social Security Office if you did not receive one with this form;) and
2. A signed statement from the physician or supplier which shows that the physician or supplier refuses to accept assignment for the bill; and
3. An itemized bill from the physician or supplier which identifies you as the person to whom the physician or supplier looks for payment.

Sign below and return this form together with the documents specified above to the address shown in the upper left portion of the form on the other side. If no carrier name and address is shown on the other side of this form request the proper addressee information from a Social Security Office.

I certify that if I receive the entire amount due, I will distribute it among other persons if they are legally entitled to it. Knowing that anyone making a false statement or representation of a material fact for use in determining the right to or the amount of Health Insurance benefits commits a crime punishable under the Federal law. I certify that the above statements are true.

If this statement has been signed by mark (X), two witnesses who know the claimant should sign below, giving their full addresses. The signature and title of a Social Security employee will suffice in lieu of signatures of two witnesses.	Name of claimant *(Please print)*	
Name	Signature of claimant *(Write in ink)* **SIGN HERE ▶**	
Address *(Number and Street, City, State and ZIP Code)*	Mailing Address *(Number and Street, P.O. Box or Route)*	
Name	City, State and ZIP Code	
Address *(Number and Street, City, State and ZIP Code)*	Date *(Month, Day and Year)*	Telephone number

If you wish assistance in completing this request, please take it to a Social Security Office. The people there will help you.
PLEASE RETURN THIS REQUEST IN THE ENCLOSED ENVELOPE.

Public reporting burden for this collection of information is estimated to average15 minutes per response, including the time for reviewing instructions, searching existing data sources, gathering and maintaining the data needed, and completing and reviewing the collection of information. Send comments regarding this burden estimate or any other aspect of this collection of information, including suggestions for reducing this burden, to HCFA, P.O. Box 26684, Baltimore, MD 21207; and to the Office of Information and Regulatory Affairs, Office of Management and Budget, Washington, D.C. 20503.

HCFA-1660 (6-81) ☆U.S. GPO: 1989-241-188/03823

Figure 6.7 Continued

COLORADO GERONTOLOGICAL SOCIETY/SENIOR HEALTH INSURANCE COUNSELING PROGRAM/P.O. BOX 18221 DENVER, CO 80218
303-333-3482

Health Insurance Claim For: ____________ Phone: ____________ Address: ____________

Medicare Claim #: ____________ Supplemental Insurance: ____________ Policy #: ____________

ALWAYS KEEP ORIGINAL PAPERWORK. SEND ONLY PHOTOCOPIES OR DUPLICATE BILLS TO OTHERS!

Date of Service	Provider or MD	Service	Charge for Service	Date sent to Medicare	Date received from Medicare	Amount Approved	Medicare Amount Paid	Patient's Balance	Assignment Accepted Yes/No	Comments	Date Sent to Supp./ by Whom	Amount/ Date Received	Check Pay to:	Patient's Remaining Balance	Awaiting Bills From Provider	Date/Amount Patient Payment	Comments/ Deductibles

Figure 6.8 Colorado Senior Health Counseling Program Record-Keeping Form

7

OTHER BENEFIT PROGRAMS

Federal, Railroad, State and Local Employees, and Veterans

FEDERAL EMPLOYEE BENEFITS

Are Federal Employees Over Age 65 Eligible for Medicare?

Some are eligible and some are not. Those who are not eligible for Medicare include civil service personnel who prior to 1983 worked for the federal government and did not pay into Social Security. (These people are not eligible unless they worked outside the federal government long enough to qualify for Social Security benefits or married a person who qualifies for benefits.) When these people retire, they are eligible for federal health benefits.

Those federal employees who as of January 1, 1983 are subject to a tax for Medicare Part A (hospital insurance) are also eligible at age 65 for Medicare.

As of January 1, 1984, all newly hired federal workers and those workers who are rehired after a separation of more than 365 days are eligible for Medicare. These workers pay into Social Security and remain part of a modified civil service retirement program. Anyone who was working for the government before January 1, 1984 can choose to pay into Social Security. Also eligible are persons who worked for the federal government but who also worked at other jobs outside the government and through this non-federal employment earned enough quarters to be eligible for Social Security and Medicare benefits.

Persons who retire from uniformed services (do not confuse these military retirees with "veterans" who are much broader segment) paid into Social Security and are entitled to Medicare. They are also eligible to receive benefits at bases and military hospitals, such as Fitzsimons Army Hospital, Bethesda Naval Hospital, etc. This group sometimes elects not to purchase Part B of Medicare since they receive health services at military bases. In an emergency or if services at the local military hospital are limited or if the hospital closes, however, veterans may need to use a civilian facility, so enrolling in Medicare and purchasing a Medicare supplement should be considered.

If Federal Retirees Are Eligible for Medicare Part A, Based on Their Own Work Record or on That of a Spouse, Should They Buy Part B?

At this time, the decision to purchase Part B should be based on retiree's finances. If they can get better coverage—and often they can—through one of the Federal Employee Plans (FEP) coordinated with Medicare Part B (in which case Medicare pays first), it is worth paying the monthly Part B premium, as well as the monthly FEP premium. Without Part B, the FEP provides only partial coverage.

It is usually less expensive for a person to downgrade coverage from an FEP high-option plan to Medicare Part B and a standard plan. Coverage situations for dependents may differ.

RAILROAD RETIREE BENEFITS

Who Are Railroad Retirees, and What Health Benefits Do They Receive at Age 65?

Persons who retired from a United States railroad company are entitled to Medicare benefits. For railroad retirees, the government contracts with The Travelers Insurance Company to process Medicare claims. These offices are located in Augusta, Georgia, and Salt Lake City, Utah. A retired railroad beneficiary's Medicare claim number begins with the letter A; the spouse with MA. A widow or widower's claim number begins with WA.

The Travelers Company, as well as the railroad companies, offers railroad retirees policies that supplement Medicare. Retirees, however, should compare prices in the marketplace before choosing railroad insurance.

After September 1, 1990, providers must submit claims to Medicare on behalf of patients. In those rare occasions when railroad retirees have to submit a Medicare claim, they should use Form G-740S, "A Patient's Request for Medicare Payment." If a railroad retiree also collects cash benefits from Social Security, the monthly premium for Medicare Part B is deducted from the railroad retirement pension check.

STATE AND LOCAL EMPLOYEE BENEFITS

Are Persons Who Retire from State and Local Employment, Such as School Teachers, Police Officers, or Public Transportation Workers, Eligible for Medicare?

Some are and some are not. Employees of state and local governments can be brought under Social Security only by means of agreements entered into by the states with the Secretary of Health and Human Services. In fact, most public employees are covered by these agreements. Some public employees have funds withheld from their salaries that go into private pension plans rather than toward Social Security. These plans usually provide health benefits for retired employees. A retiree also may have earned enough Social Security quarters to be eligible for Medicare by virtue of some other employment.

Note: Congress changed the law and extended Medicare to all state and local government employees who were hired after April 1986. Employees and their employers pay employment taxes that go into the Medicare Hospital (Part A) Trust Fund, so they may be eligible for Medicare when they turn age 65.

VETERANS' BENEFITS

Who Is Considered a Veteran?

Generally, a veteran is any person who has been honorably discharged from the armed forces (army, navy, air force) and who, after September 1980, also served at least 24 months in the armed forces. There are approximately 27,000,000 veterans in the United States. Most states have a Division of Veterans Affairs and local county veterans service offices who can assist residents.

Are Retired Men and Women Who Served in the Military Services Eligible for Both Veterans' Benefits and Medicare?

Yes, those persons eligible for Social Security benefits are, at age 65, automatically entitled to enroll in

Medicare. Any veteran is also eligible for health care through the Veterans Administration (VA). However, services received at VA medical centers or clinics will not be paid for by Medicare, nor will most services at a non-VA hospital or by a non-VA physician, even when referred and authorized by the Veterans Administration.

Which Veterans Are Eligible for VA Hospital and Nursing Home Care?

Although free inpatient hospital and nursing home care services are available to all veterans, the intent of recent laws is to ensure that VA care is provided first to veterans with service-connected disabilities and to lower income veterans. Legislation in 1986 established three categories of eligibility for VA health care, along with eligibility assessments in each category.

Category A

Includes veterans with service-connected disabilities, former prisoners of war, veterans receiving VA pensions, etc. Others in Category "A" include those who have a nonservice-connected disability, *and* meet the eligibility assessment ($17,240 or below per year for a single veteran in 1990 and $20,688 if married. These figures are adjusted annually in February). The VA *will* provide hospital care and *may* provide nursing home and outpatient care if space and resources are available.

Category B

Includes veterans with nonservice-connected disabilities who have higher income levels than Category A. The VA may provide hospital, outpatient, and nursing home care if space and resources are available. In practice, people in this category are not currently receiving benefits due to budget restrictions.

Category C

Includes veterans with nonservice-connected disabilities and some higher income levels than Category B allows. The VA may provide care if space and resources are available. Veterans in Category C must pay the VA a copayment for their care. In practice, people in this category are not currently receiving benefits due to budget restrictions.

What Types of Medical Care Are Available Through the VA System?

Outpatient/Ambulatory Care

Medical services are provided to eligible veterans if resources and facilities are available. It is difficult to understand the restrictions, so it is advisable to seek care and let the VA decide if a person is eligible. Generally, services are provided without limitations to veterans with service-connected disability ratings of 50% or more. Also, care may be available to those meeting income eligibility of $11,409 or less for a single veteran and $13,620 for a couple in 1991. Some veterans are assessed a copayment for services.

Outpatient dental treatment, alcohol and drug dependence treatment, and prosthetic appliances are available to eligible veterans. Prescription drugs are available to service-connected veterans with no copayment; nonservice-connected veterans pay $2 per prescription.

Note: Emergency services are not always available at VA facilities. If a veteran is admitted to a private hospital in an emergency, the VA determines whether to authorize payment for the ambulance and for the hospital.

Inpatient Hospital Care

Priority is given to Category A veterans who need hospitalization for service-connected diseases or injuries.

Nursing Home Care

Veterans may also qualify for care at VA expense in a federal VA nursing facility or a state Veterans Home. State Veterans Homes are administered by the individual states; however, since they are subsidized by the Department of Veterans Affairs they cost less than private nursing homes. However, as with most hospital admissions, priorities apply. Veterans in Category A who have service-connected disabilities have priority for admission.

Note: Many wartime veterans who need nursing-home care are eligible for nonservice-connected pensions with "Aid and Attendance" benefits (an add-on benefit to the pension of certain eligible veterans in need of nursing home care). These veterans are eligible for the pensions because the cost of nursing home care is deducted when calculating total income and resources. Many widows are also eligible for these pensions. Contact your State Veterans Affairs office or service organization (Disabled American Veterans) or the federal Department of Veterans Affairs for more details.

8

THE MEDICAID PROGRAM

WHAT IS MEDICAID?

Medicaid (Title XIX of the Social Security Act) is a federal/state program (unlike Medicare, which is entirely federal) that provides certain needy persons with financial assistance for their health care. Payment for medical services is made directly to the care providers by the agency charged with administration of the Medicaid program in each state. To receive Medicaid benefits, a person must be in a low-income category and meet specific eligibility requirements.

Medicaid is administered by the Health Care Financing Administration within the U.S. Department of Health and Human Services. Funding for the program comes, in part, from the federal government and from the individual states. Contact your state or local social service agency or medical assistance (Medicaid) office for more information on Medicaid.

The Medicaid program varies from state to state in terms of the programs the state elects to provide for its residents. Eligibility requirements for maximum income and allowable assets also vary from state to state. However, *all* states *must* provide assistance to needy persons who fall into certain categories such as blind, disabled, aged (65 or older), and those eligible for Aid to Families with Dependent Children (AFDC).

What Are the National Poverty Level Figures for Persons Over Age 65?

These figures are revised annually in February. The 1991 figures are:

Individual income limit: $551.67 per month or $6,620.00 per year

Couple's income limit: $740.00 per month or $8,880.00 per year

What Are the Medicaid Eligibility Categories for People Over Age 60?

A person on Medicare whose income falls below a certain income level can receive Medicaid assistance. Medicaid acts as a supplement to Medicare, doing away with the need to purchase a Medicare supplemental insurance policy. Also, Medicaid will pay the monthly Medicare Part B premium, deductibles, and coinsurance. Below are some of the Medicaid eligibility categories for people over age 60.

Blind, Disabled, and Aged Persons (Over 65)

People in this category who fall below a certain income and asset limit are eligible for Supplemental Security Income (SSI), a federal income assistance program. In most states if a person is receiving SSI, he or she is automatically eligible for Medicaid. In 1991, to qualify for SSI, income must be $407 per month or less for a single person and $610 per month for a couple. (These figures do not take into account adjustments for earned versus unearned income, etc.) Those resources or assets that count toward eligibility (see "Countable Resources") cannot exceed more than $2,000 for an individual and $3,000 for a couple.

Optional State Supplement Programs

Some persons age 60 or over who fall below certain income and asset limits may be eligible for state programs that supplement their income and make them automatically eligible for their state's Medicaid program.

Medically Needy Programs

Some states (using federal and state funds) provide assistance to persons who are "medically needy," that is, those who would not normally qualify for Medicaid but whose medial expenses are higher than their monthly income. Thirty-five states presently use state Medicaid funds to provide assistance to persons in a nursing home whose monthly income exceeds Medicaid limits but who cannot afford the cost of nursing home care.

Institutionalization

A person may also become eligible for Medicaid if he or she is institutionalized in a nursing home or hospital for at least 30 consecutive days and has income and assets below a certain level. In 1991 in some states the institutionalized person's income must be below $1,221 per month. Countable resources must be spent down to $2,000 before Medicaid will pay for care.

Qualified Medicare Beneficiary (QMB)

In all states certain low-income Medicare beneficiaries over 65 and certain low-income persons receiving Medicare because of a disability may qualify for Medicaid under the Qualified Medicare Beneficiary (QMB) benefit. In 1991, states are required to pay ("buy in") Medicare Part B premiums, deductibles, and coinsurance for Qualified Medicare Beneficiaries who have income at or below 100% of the national poverty level rate. The maximum income varies from state to state. Countable resources cannot exceed $4,000 for a single person and $6,000 for a married couple. States are also required to pay Part A premiums for certain working disabled people with incomes up to 200% of the poverty level, although those with incomes above 150% of poverty may be required to contribute to the premium.

Does Medicaid Cover Persons in a Nursing Home?

In most states people confined to a nursing home for 30 consecutive days whose monthly income falls below 300% of the annual Supplemental Security Income limit ($1,221 per month or less in 1991) and who meet their state's resource limits are eligible for Medicaid, which will pay for their care in a nursing home. Residents of some states may only have to meet their state's resource limits to be eligible for Medicaid.

What Happens to People's Resources Once They Qualify for Medicaid Assistance in a Nursing Home?

Unmarried people must deplete most of their countable resources or assets (to $2,000) in order to have the Medicaid program pay for their stay. However, as a result of the Medicaid "spousal protection" portion of the 1988 Catastrophic Coverage Act, effective September 30, 1989, the "community" spouse (person living at home) is permitted to maintain a minimum monthly income that is a specified percentage of poverty level as determined by the state (but not less than $856/month). These figures change annually. The community spouse is also allowed to retain a minimum of $13,250 of the couple's resources. Some states have adopted a maximum monthly income protection limit (approximately $1,600 per month) and maximum asset protection (approximately $66,000).

The impact of the new law means that some of the institutionalized spouse's income may be directed back to the community spouse to bring that person's income up to a minimum level and, also, all their resources do not have to be used to pay for the nursing home stay.

Note: This law only applies to married couples in a situation where the institutionalized spouse is eligible for Medicaid in a nursing home.

Example: Assume that Peter and his wife, Rosa, have $26,500 in a bank account. Peter is admitted to a nursing home after September 30, 1989 and is eligible for Medicaid. Rosa, as the community spouse, is allowed to divide their "countable resources" in half and retain a minimum of $13,250 in assets. Peter, as the institutionalized spouse, has to "spend down" his $13,250 share of their resources to $2,000, but Rosa does not have to spend her share toward Peter's nursing home costs. This will protect Rosa from having to spend all their resources.

The Utah Gap

The problem of impoverishment is not solved, however, for many people. In some states, a person may fall into the "Utah gap," that is, a situation in which a person's monthly income is over the income limit for Medicaid eligibility. This person will not be eligible for Medicaid even when resources are depleted and will have to pay for his or her own care in a nursing home. Since the average nursing home costs between $2,100 and $2,400 a month, the community spouse and, perhaps, other family members will undoubtedly try to assist with paying the cost of the spouse's care and may also become impoverished. (In Colorado, which is a "Utah gap" state, the validity of *Medicaid Secondary Needs Trusts* is being tested in the courts for certain incapacitated patients who have exhausted most of their resources. Through this instrument the institutionalized patient is paid a monthly income from his trust that is $20 under the eligibility limit so as to qualify him for Medicaid.)

Are People Who Are Receiving Medicare Benefits Also Eligible for Medicaid?

Yes, people who have Medicare and who meet the low-income and resource requirements may be eligible for Medicaid. The patient may have to pay a small copayment for some services, such as doctor visits and prescription drugs. Providers must accept Medicare assignment and must submit claims to Medicare first and then to Medicaid. Health care providers do not have to serve Medicaid patients.

Note: A person who is receiving Medicare benefits and who is also receiving Medicaid benefits should not purchase a Medicare supplement. Only in rare situations would it be prudent to retain a Medicare supplement; for example, persons paying a small monthly amount for an employer group coverage plan that does not allow them to re-enroll if they drop this plan would want to have a Medicare supplement. Persons whose income is expected to increase due to inheritance or V. A. benefits would also want a Medicare supplement in case this increase in income exceeds the Medicaid maximum income level and makes them ineligible for Medicaid.

How Do You Apply for Medicaid?

1. Complete an initial application
2. Make an appointment for the interview to review the application
3. Bring the following to the interview

- Proof of age/citizenship
- Proof of assets
- Proof of income
- Proof of life insurance, health insurance, burial policies
- Medicare and Social Security cards

Note: Eligibility for Medicaid must be reconsidered periodically, usually every 6 to 12 months.

What Does Medicaid Consider "Income"?

Income includes wages, social Security cash benefits, other pensions or retirement benefits, unemployment insurance, gifts, interest, dividends, etc. Income from pensions and individual retirement accounts (IRAs) are assumed to belong to that member of a married couple who earned or owns the benefit.

What Are "Countable Resources" or "Nonexempt Resources" in Terms of Medicaid Eligibility?

Note: Check specific regulations in your state.

Assets that count toward Medicaid eligibility include the following.

- Cash
- Certificates of deposit
- Checking and savings accounts
- Money market accounts
- Stocks and bonds
- Real estate
- Face value (amount paid at death) of whole life insurance policies over $1,500

Assets that *are exempt* include the following.

- House (depends on state regulations) If you, your spouse, or a dependent child reside in it, or if there is an intent to return home.
- Car (no dollar limit if equipped for handicapped, or if used for work or to seek medical treatment, otherwise $4,500 limit)
- Personal belongings (up to $2,000 limit)
- Irrevocable burial/funeral policy or revocable burial /funeral and face value of a life insurance not to exceed $1,500
- Life insurance policies are exempt up to a face value of $1,500 (Up to $1,500 of cash surrender value is exempt on face values over $1,500.) Term life insurance is excluded, since you must die to collect.

Irrevocable trusts are not exempt. Also, certificates of deposits that are in child's and parent's name jointly are most often considered the parent's and can be split only in proportion to cash contributions made by the child.

You cannot transfer property just to be eligible for Medicaid. You must sell property for fair market value and then spend down the assets if they are above the Medicaid guidelines. If property or assets are transferred, there is a time period during which the person is not eligible for Medicaid. If the transfer was made after July 1, 1988, there is a 30-month penalty.

What Kinds of Medical Services Can an Older Adult Receive on Medicaid?

All states presently have a Medicaid program although programs vary from state to state. In order to receive federal funding a state's Medicaid program must offer certain basic medical services. These basic medical services include the following.

- Inpatient hospital services
- Outpatient hospital services
- Lab and X ray
- Physician services
- Home health care
- Skilled nursing facility care for adults
- Family planning
- Rural health clinics
- EPSDT services for people under age 21 (early periodic screening, diagnostic, and treatment services)

In addition to basic medical services, states may choose to provide additional coverage such as prescription drugs, intermediate and custodial nursing home coverage, transportation, dental care, eyeglasses, hearing aids, vision screening, prosthetic devices, durable medical equipment, mental health services, and certain therapies.

GLOSSARY

A

Actual Charge The original fee charged by the health care provider.

Acute Care Care provided for a serious medical problem needing immediate attention.

Allowable Charge The maximum amount a third party (insurance company) will allow when reimbursing for a service. Also, Medicare's maximum amount of reimbursement on a claim as determined by their guidelines (*See also* Approved and Reasonable).

Ambulatory Care Outpatient health care services.

Ancillary Services X ray, laboratory, and hospital services other than room and board.

Approved Charge Medicare's maximum amount of reimbursement on a claim as determined by their guideline (*See Also* Allowable and Reasonable).

Assignment Provider agrees to accept as full payment whatever charge Medicare "approves" as reasonable, although coinsurance and deductibles are still owed.

B

Balance Billing On an unassigned claim, this is the amount of money over and above what Medicare approves, up to the provider's actual charge (Also called the "excess").

Beneficiary A person who receives benefits.

Benefit Maximum Limits the dollar amount for a benefit or a time period for which the policy will pay.

Biologicals Substances such as whole blood, hemophilia clotting factors, tetanus antitoxins, heparin (used in a home dialysis system, which is a medical supply), botulin antitoxin, vaccines, tumor chemotherapy agent (goes into an infusion pump, which is a medical supply), hepatitis vaccine.

Black Lung Disease (pneumoconiosis) Lung disease related to work in coal mines. The Federal Coal Mine Health and Safety Act provides for certain benefits for victims of this disease.

Blue Cross/Blue Shield Association A nationwide federation of local, nonprofit insurance organizations that contracts with hospitals and other health care providers to make payments for health care services to subscribers.

Buy-In A program in which a state's Medicaid program pays Medicare premiums, deductibles, and coinsurance for certain eligible low-income people.

C

Calendar Year Refers to period of time between January 1 and December 31.

Carrier A private insurance company that is under contract with the Health Care Financing Administration to process Part B Medicare claims.

Carve Out A supplement to Medicare that provides retired employees with the same health care benefits as active employees, minus what Medicare pays.

Catastrophic Coverage Act of 1988 Law that expanded Medicare benefits. The Medicare portion was repealed in 1989.

Catastrophic Health Insurance A type of insurance policy that provides protection against the high cost of treating severe or lengthy illnesses or disabilities. These policies generally cover a percentage of medical expenses above a deductible amount—which is the policyholder's responsibility—up to a certain maximum amount.

Claim A bill requesting that medical services be paid for by Medicare or by some other insurance company.

Coinsurance A specified amount of money that an insurance policyholder shares on a claim.

Competitive Medical Plan (CMP) A type of prepayment health plan that is similar to a health maintenance organization.

Consolidated Omnibus Budget Reconciliation Act (COBRA) Legislation Legislation passed in 1986 giving workers who are no longer employed due to retirement or termination the option of purchasing employee group health insurance for 18 months.

Conversion Privilege In group health insurance, the right of an insured person, upon termination of the group insurance, to change group coverage to individual coverage without a health screening. Group policies often terminate when employment or membership in a group ends.

Coordination of Benefits Wording in an insurance policy stating that the policy will not pay a covered expense on a claim if another policy pays it. Or it may pay part of the costs, not to exceed the total actual cost (100%) of the service. Coordination of benefits prevents duplication of payments to a policyholder who is insured under more than one policy.

Copayment (Cost Sharing) The insured person pays a specified fixed amount per unit of service, such as $5 for an office visit, at the time of service.

Covered Services Health care services by Medicare-approved providers for which Medicare will partially pay.

Current Procedural Terminology (CPT) A system of terms and codes developed by the American Medical Association that is used for describing, coding, and reporting medical services and procedures.

Custodial Care A level of nonmedical care that provides assistance with the activities of daily living. Does not require licensed professionals, such as a physician or a registered nurse.

Customary Charge The amount that a physician or supplier most frequently charges for a particular service or supply.

D

Deductible An amount of money that a person must pay before his or her insurance begins to pay on a claim.

Department of Health and Human Services (DHHS) An executive department of the federal government that has ultimate authority for the Medicare and Medicaid programs.

Diagnosis Related Groups (DRG) Refers to categories of illnesses that are divided into 490 groups, one of which is assigned to a Medicare patient upon discharge from a hospital. The hospital is reimbursed a fixed amount based on the DRG code for the patient.

Discharge Planner A person who is employed by a hospital to assist patients in planning and meeting their post hospital health care needs.

Durable Medical Equipment (DME) Equipment that can be used repeatedly for medical purposes by an ill or injured person, such as, wheelchairs, crutches, walkers, oxygen, etc.

E

Electronic Media Claim (EMC) The electronic transmittal of claims information between the provider and Medicare or Medicaid (Also called "electronic billing").

Elimination Period This refers to a period of time when a policy is not in full force and the patient is responsible for medical costs as in long-term care insurance.

End Stage Renal Disease (ESRD) A permanent and irreversible kidney disease that requires dialysis or kidney transplant to maintain life. This disease is covered by Medicare.

Excess On an unassigned claim, this is the amount of money over and above what Medicare approves, up to the provider's actual charge (Also called "balance billing").

Exclusion Refers to something for which the policy will not pay.

Extended Care The skilled care that often follows an acute illness and may be received either in a skilled nursing facility or hospital. Now commonly known as "skilled nursing facility" benefits.

F

First Dollar Coverage Insurance policy pays the first dollar of covered expense incurred by the policyholder.

G

General Enrollment Period The annual period from January 1 through March 31 in which a person may enroll in Medicare Part B; benefits take effect on July 1.

Guaranteed Renewable Guarantees that a person can retain an insurance policy up to the age specified in the policy (often 65). Medicare supplements are often guaranteed renewable for life. Premiums can only be raised if they are raised for all beneficiaries in a specified state, for example.

H

Health Care Financing Administration (HCFA) The agency in the Department of Health and Human Services that administers Medicare and Medicaid.

Health Maintenance Organization (HMO) A prepayment health care plan.

Home Health Agency A public or private agency that provides skilled and other health care services in the home.

Home Health Aide A person who under the supervision of a skilled nurse provides personal care assistance (eating, bathing, etc.) to persons in their home.

Hospice Programs designed for caring for the terminally ill and employing specially trained caregivers.

Hospital Insurance Another term for Part A of Medicare.

I

Initial Enrollment Period The 7 months surrounding a person's 65th birth month in which he or she may enroll in Medicare.

Inpatient A person who is "admitted" to a hospital or nursing home and receives medical services while staying overnight.

Insurance Pool An organization of insurers or reinsurers that share or pool particular types of risks. The risk of high loss by any particular insurance company is transferred to the group as a whole with premiums, losses, and expenses shared in agreed amounts.

Intermediary or **Fiscal Intermediary** A private insurance company that is under contract with the Health Care Financing Administration to handle Part A claims processing.

Intermediate Care Facility (ICF) Nursing homes that are not licensed to provide skilled care. Medicare does not pay for care in an ICF even though they may provide some skilled services.

L

Lifetime Maximum The maximum dollar amount an insurance policy will pay during a person's lifetime.

Long-term Care Health and/or personal care services required by persons in an institution or at home over a long period of time.

M

Mail Order Insurance Life, accident, health, or disability insurance secured by mail; usually requires no physical exam, only a statement of health status completed by the insured.

Major Medical Insurance policy that is designed to help pay for very expensive illnesses; differs from first-dollar coverage. Usually it has a high deductible and a high lifetime maximum.

Mammogram X ray of the breast to diagnose breast cancer.

Medicaid Title XIX of the Social Security Act. Medical assistance to low-income persons who fall into certain specific categories. The program is funded by the federal government and the individual states.

Medical Insurance Another term for Part B of Medicare.

Medicare Title XVIII of the Social Security Act. Federal health insurance program for people age 65 and older who are eligible for Social Security cash benefits.

Medigap These are the services that Medicare does not cover or that require a coinsurance or deductible might pay. Medigap insurance refers to the private health insurance designed to supplement Medicare.

N

National Association of Insurance Commissioners (NAIC) The organization that prepares model provisions and guidelines for insurance companies and state legislatures.

Nursing Home A place where persons reside who need medical care and/or personal assistance with the activities of daily living.

O

Occupational Therapy Activities designed to improve the functioning of physically and/or mentally disabled persons.

Open Enrollment A period when new subscribers may elect to enroll in a health insurance plan or health maintenance organization.

Outliers Unusually long inpatient stays or expensive Medicare cases that result in additional diagnosis related group payments to providers.

Out-of-pocket Expenses Costs borne directly by the patient.

Outpatient Refers to services received while not staying overnight at a hospital or other facility.

P

Part A Medicare's "Hospital Insurance" (HI) provides coverage for inpatient hospital stays, inpatient stays in a skilled nursing facility, home health care, and hospice care.

Part B Medicare's "Medical Insurance" or "Supplemental Medical Insurance" (SMI) provides coverage for physician's services and other outpatient services.

Participating A "participating" provider is one who signs a contract with Medicare or a private insurance company and agrees to accept Medicare's or the insurance company's approved amount as the maximum amount that provider will charge the patient. Participating providers "accept assignment."

Pathology Services Diagnosis of disease by studying tissues removed during operations and postmortem exams. Includes anatomic, cellular, hematological, and cytological pathology.

Peer Review Organization (PRO) A physician-sponsored, nongovernmental organization of health professionals in each state under contract to the federal government to review appropriateness and quality of hospital treatment of Medicare patients before, during, and after their stay.

Personal Comfort Items Items such as a television, telephone, etc. provided in hospitals and other health care facilities.

Preexisting Condition A health problem that exists at the time a person purchases an insurance policy. That health problem may be excluded from coverage for a certain period of time as noted in the policy. Even if a person has not visited a physician for a long period of time, if he or she is still taking a prescription drug for any condition, that condition is considered "preexisting."

Preferred Provider Organization (PPO) An organization that contracts with a third party payer such as an insurer, a union trust fund, or self-insured employer to furnish health care services at lower than usual fees in return for prompt payment and an increased number of patients.

Premium Money paid for an insurance contract that is paid monthly, quarterly, semi-annually, or annually.

Prevailing Charge A specified percentile of the "customary charge" for a designated service by all physicians in a certain region. This is usually the maximum charge Medicare can approve for any item or service.

Primary Care (Basic Health Care) Primary health care providers assume ongoing responsibility for the patient in both health maintenance and the treatment of an illness.

Prospective Payment System A system of reimbursing hospitals for Medicare patients' services based on a predetermined amount related to the principal diagnosis of the patient.

Prosthetic Device Device that replaces a body part such as artificial limbs, or lens implants.

Provider Someone who provides medical services or supplies such as a physician, hospital, X-ray company, home health agency, or pharmacy.

Q

Qualified Medicare Beneficiary A special category of low-income elderly and disabled Medicare beneficiaries who are eligible for Medicaid.

R

Radiology Services X rays and related diagnostic tests such as angiograms, pyelograms, and myelograms.

Railroad Retiree Person who worked for a railroad company and is entitled to benefits at retirement (includes Medicare).

Reasonable Charge Medicare's maximum amount of reimbursement on a claim as determined by Medicare guidelines. Medicare usually pays 80% of the reasonable charge (*See also* Approved and Allowable).

Relative Value Scale (RVS) A listing of physician services using units that indicate their relative value. The RVS will be used to establish a physician's fee schedule.

Rider A document that modifies the insurance policy coverage, either by expanding or decreasing benefits.

S

Skilled Care A level of care that requires the services of a registered nurse and/or professional therapist, such as a physical or speech therapist, under supervision of a physician.

Skilled Nursing Facility A health care facility that is specially licensed and staffed to provide nursing, rehabilitation, and other services.

Social Security Act Legislation enacted in 1935, along with other related laws, that provides for the material needs of individuals and families, protects aged and disabled persons against the expenses of illnesses that could otherwise exhaust their savings (Medicare), "keeps families together, and gives children the opportunity to grow up in good health and security." Social Security programs include retirement insurance, survivors insurance, disability insurance, Medicare, black lung benefits, supplemental security income, unemployment insurance, and public assistance and welfare services such as aid to needy families with children, medical assistance (Medicaid), maternal and child health services, child support enforcement, family and child welfare services, food stamps, and energy assistance. Some of these programs are operated solely by the federal government and some are operated in cooperation with the individual states.

Supplemental Health Insurance Insurance that may cover the Medicare coinsurance, deductibles, and noncovered services not covered by Medicare benefits.

Supplemental Security (SSI) Income A federal income-assistance program for low-income aged, blind, and disabled persons.

T

Tax Liability The amount of tax a person owes.

U

Unassigned Claim A medical claim for which the provider's actual billed charge is due. Payment is made to the insured person rather than to the provider.

Underwriting The statistical process by which an insurer establishes and assumes risks according to insurability.

United States Included are the 50 states, the District of Columbia, Guam, American Samoa, American Virgin Islands, Puerto Rico, and the Northern Mariana Islands.

Usual, Reasonable, Customary Charges (UCR) In insurance terminology this is the maximum amount a company will pay on a claim as determined by their guidelines (similar to Medicare's "approved charge").

Utilization Review Committee A committee in a health care facility (hospital, nursing home) that evaluates the necessity, appropriateness, and efficiency of the use of medical services, procedures, and facilities.

Utilization Screens These are the prudent amounts of medical services permitted in a given time period, as determined by the Medicare contractor.

W

Waiting Period Refers to the period of time a person will have to pay for services before benefits are active. An insurance policy is not in full force during this period.

INDEX

I

L

M

N

O

P

Q

R

S

T

U

V

W

X

ABOUT THE AUTHORS

Leonard H. Hellman is a licensed attorney and physician specializing in geriatrics. In 1979, he implemented an innovative hospital-based outpatient clinic for seniors that provided comprehensive, case-managed health care. He is Cofounder and Medical Director of GeriMed of America, Inc., a consulting and management company that assists U.S. and Canadian hospitals with geriatric services, and he is past President of the Colorado Gerontological Society. He also serves as Medical Director to a number of nursing homes.

A graduate of New York University Law School and Mount Sinai School of Medicine in New York, he received his graduate medical training at Mary Hitchcock Hospital, Dartmouth Medical Center in Hanover, New Hampshire. He lectures extensively on medical, social, and legal issues of aging and is a frequent keynote speaker on "Humor in Aging."

Susan Hellman is Founder and Director of Colorado's *Senior Health Insurance Counseling Program (SHIC-P)*, where she trains and supervises counselors in a volunteer program that provides assistance to older adults who are having problems dealing with Medicare. She is a graduate of Cornell University and holds an MA from Columbia University.

She frequently lectures and writes articles on the subject of Medicare and retirement health insurance and teaches seminars to professionals in the community including a college course entitled, "Tackling Medicare Paperwork." She authors an annual "Shopper's Guide to Senior Health Insurance" and often appears as a guest expert on local senior-oriented radio and television shows. She also serves on the Medicare Regulations Advisory Committee at the Colorado Division of Insurance and on a Senior Coalition Committee at the Colorado Medical Society.

Practice Behaviors Workbook

Understanding Human Behavior in the Social Environment

NINTH EDITION

Charles H. Zastrow
George Williams College of Aurura University

Karen K. Kirst-Ashman
University of Wisconsin, Whitewater

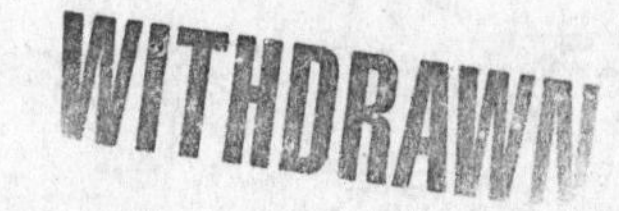

Prepared by

Vicki Vogel
University of Wisconsin, Whitewater

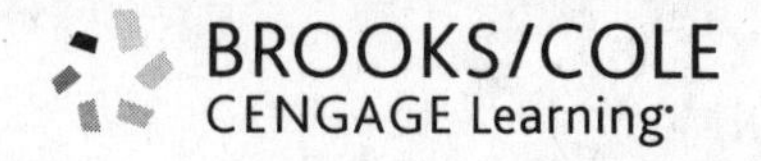

Australia • Brazil • Japan • Korea • Mexico • Singapore • Spain • United Kingdom • United States

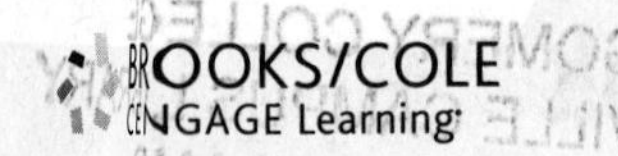

For product information and technology assistance, contact us at **Cengage Learning Customer & Sales Support, 1-800-354-9706**

For permission to use material from this text or product, submit all requests online at **www.cengage.com/permissions**
Further permissions questions can be emailed to **permissionrequest@cengage.com**

ISBN-13: 978-1-133-35424-6
ISBN-10: 1-133-35424-6

Brooks/Cole
20 Davis Drive
Belmont, CA 94002-3098
USA

Cengage Learning is a leading provider of customized learning solutions with office locations around the globe, including Singapore, the United Kingdom, Australia, Mexico, Brazil, and Japan. Locate your local office at: **www.cengage.com/global**

Cengage Learning products are represented in Canada by Nelson Education, Ltd.

To learn more about Brooks/Cole, visit **www.cengage.com/brookscole**

Purchase any of our products at your local college store or at our preferred online store **www.cengagebrain.com**

Printed in the United States of America
1 2 3 4 5 6 7 16 15 14 13 12

Contents

NOTE TO INSTRUCTORS:
Commentary to Instructors is located in the Instructors Manual and includes information/ answers for some of the exercises found in this Workbook.

Empowerment Series

Dear Social Work Student,

Welcome to *Competencies/Practice Behaviors Workbook* for Zastrow/Kirst-Ashman's *Understanding Human Behavior and the Social Environment*, 9e. Throughout your course you will acquire a great deal of new knowledge, including an introduction to new theories, informative research, and practical skills like critical thinking skills and frameworks for appreciating and overcoming challenges. All of the knowledge you gain will offer you a deeper, richer understanding of social work. Used in conjunction with your text and other resources, the *Competencies/Practice Behaviors Workbook* presents you with Practice Exercises that will teach you how to transform your new knowledge into social work Practice Behaviors.

About Competence and Practice Behaviors

In social work, the words Competence and Practice Behavior have a unique meaning beyond the typical dictionary definitions. "Competence" in the usual sense means that a person possesses suitable skills and abilities to do a specific task. A competent baseball player must move quickly, catch, throw, and play as part of a team. They also have to think quickly, understand the rules of the game, and be knowledgeable of their environment. In the same way, a competent social worker should be able to do a number of job-related duties, think critically, and understand the context of their work. The Council on Social Work Education (CSWE) has defined specific Core Competency areas for all social work students, and their corresponding Practice Behaviors as follows:

Competencies and Practice Behaviors	
2.1.1:	**Identify as a Professional Social Worker and Conduct Oneself Accordingly**
a.	Advocate for client access to the services of social work
b.	Practice personal reflection and self-correction to assure continual professional development
c.	Attend to professional roles and boundaries
d.	Demonstrate professional demeanor in behavior, appearance, and communication
e.	Engage in career-long learning
f.	Use supervision and consultation
2.1.2:	**Apply Social Work Ethical Principles to Guide Professional Practice**
a.	Recognize and manage personal values in a way that allows professional values to guide practice
b.	Make ethical decisions by applying standards of the National Association of Social Workers Code of Ethics and, as applicable, of the International Federation of Social Workers/ International Association of Schools of Social Work Ethics in Social Work, Statement of Principles
c.	Tolerate ambiguity in resolving ethical conflicts
d.	Apply strategies of ethical reasoning to arrive at principled decisions

2.1.3:	**Apply Critical Thinking to Inform and Communicate Professional Judgments**
a.	Distinguish, appraise, and integrate multiple sources of knowledge, including research-based knowledge and practice wisdom
b.	Analyze models of assessment, prevention, intervention, and evaluation
c.	Demonstrate effective oral and written communication in working with individuals, families, groups, organizations, communities, and colleagues
2.1.4:	**Engage Diversity and Difference in Practice**
a.	Recognize the extent to which a culture's structures and values may oppress, marginalize, alienate, or create or enhance privilege and power
b.	Gain sufficient self-awareness to eliminate the influence of personal biases and values in working with diverse groups
c.	Recognize and communicate their understanding of the importance of difference in shaping life experiences
d.	View themselves as learners and engage those with whom they work as informants
2.1.5:	**Advance Human Rights and Social and Economic Justice**
a.	Understand the forms and mechanisms of oppression and discrimination
b.	Advocate for human rights and social and economic justice
c.	Engage in practices that advance social and economic justice
2.1.6:	**Engage in Research-Informed Practice and Practice-Informed Research**
a.	Use practice experience to inform scientific inquiry
b.	Use research evidence to inform practice
2.1.7:	**Apply Knowledge of Human Behavior and the Social Environment**
a.	Utilize conceptual frameworks to guide the processes of assessment, intervention, and evaluation
b.	Critique and apply knowledge to understand person and environment
2.1.8:	**Engage in Policy Practice to Advance Social and Economic Well-Being and to Deliver Effective Social Work Services**
a.	Analyze, formulate, and advocate for policies that advance social well-being
b.	Collaborate with colleagues and clients for effective policy action
2.1.9:	**Respond to Contexts that Shape Practice**
a.	Continuously discover, appraise, and attend to changing locales, populations, scientific and technological developments, and emerging societal trends to provide relevant services
b.	Provide leadership in promoting sustainable changes in service delivery and practice to improve the quality of social services
2.1.10:	**Engage, Assess, Intervene, and Evaluate with Individuals, Families, Groups, Organizations and Communities**
a.	Substantively and affectively prepare for action with individuals, families, groups, organizations, and communities
b.	Use empathy and other interpersonal skills
c.	Develop a mutually agreed-on focus of work and desired outcomes
d.	Collect, organize, and interpret client data
e.	Assess client strengths and limitations
f.	Develop mutually agreed-on intervention goals and objectives
g.	Select appropriate intervention strategies
h.	Initiate actions to achieve organizational goals
i.	Implement prevention interventions that enhance client capacities
j.	Help clients resolve problems

k.	Negotiate, mediate, and advocate for clients
l.	Facilitate transitions and endings
m.	Critically analyze, monitor, and evaluate interventions

Each of the Exercises in the *Competencies/Practice Behaviors Workbook* will focus on learning and applying social work Practice Behaviors. While every Exercise will not ask you to apply Competencies or Practice Behaviors from every Core Competency area, by the time you finish your course you will have practiced many and gained a better working knowledge of how social work is done. The goal, shared by your professors, your program, the authors of this text, and by Brooks/Cole, Cengage Learning Social Work team, is that by the end of your curriculum you will have honed your Practice Behaviors in all of the Core Competency areas into a skill set that empowers you to work effectively as a professional social worker.

Assessing Competence: Partnering with Your Instructor and Peer Evaluator

As described above, the Council on Social Work Education clearly defines the Competencies and Practice Behaviors that a social work student should be trained to employ. Therefore, the grading rubric that comes at the end of every chapter of the *Competencies/Practice Behaviors Workbook* is adapted from Competencies and Practice Behaviors defined by CSWE (see the table above). To assess your competence during your course, we recommend you partner with a peer(s) who can act as your course "evaluator(s)" to genuinely assess both your written assignments and your role-plays; be sure to ask your professor to comment on and approve the assessments once they are completed by you and your Evaluator. It is our hope that partnering with your classmates in this way will familiarize you with the unique learning opportunity you will have in your Field Experience – the signature pedagogy of social work education. There you will apply all of your knowledge and skills under the supervision of your Field Instructor and Field Liaison before completing your required curriculum.

As always, we thank you for your commitment to education and to the profession. Enjoy your course, and *feel empowered to help others*!

Sincerely,

Charles Zastrow
Karen K. Kirst-Ashman
Vicki Vogel
Your Cengage Learning Social Work Team

Chapter 1
Introduction to Human Behavior and the Social Environment

Competencies/Practice Behaviors Exercise 1.1
This Is Your Life

Focus Competencies or Practice Behaviors:

- EP 2.1.1b Practice personal reflection and self-correction to assure continual professional development
- EP 2.1.4c Recognize and communicate their understanding of the importance of difference in shaping life experiences

A. Brief Description

In this exercise, you are asked to create a symbolic representation of major positive and negative events in your life.

B. Objectives

You will:

1. Identify normal life events.
2. Develop a perspective on the types of issues and simulations that will be examined throughout the course.
3. Examine the effects of various life events and relate them to the ways that similar life events may affect clients.

C. Procedure

1. Take a few moments to reflect on the most memorable occasions in your life. Think about the most positive happenings. These may include happy occasions, special activities, awards, achievements, special relationships, or graduations. Then focus on some of the major negative happenings. These might include illnesses, deaths, accidents, job losses, or significant disappointments.
2. Break into small groups of four to six. You may join any group you wish, but the groups should be the appropriate size.
3. Share as many of the positive and negative happenings in your life as you choose. Focus on the effects of these happenings on your life. You will have approximately 10 minutes for the small-group discussion.
4. After you finish your discussion, have a representative summarize some of the happenings discussed in the group and share them with the entire class.
5. As a take-home assignment, create a symbolic picture of your life. Incorporate the major positive and negative happenings. Anything you feel is too personal to share should either be excluded from the life picture or stated in vague, general terms. You may be as creative as you like in illustrating your life. Examples of different types of formats include: a line or bar graph illustrating various highs and lows; a fan that is divided into different life stages and has different colors that portray positive and negative times; a piano keyboard on which the white keys reflect positive times and the dark keys refer to negative ones; a time chart with magazine cut-outs to emphasize various life events.

The projects will not be evaluated for artistic ability but rather on such elements as depth of insight, creativity, amount of detail, and completeness. Regardless of the format, specific information needs to be clearly incorporated.

Competencies/Practice Behaviors Exercise 1.2
Social History Assignment

Focus Competencies or Practice Behaviors:

- EP 2.1.3c Demonstrate effective oral and written communication in working with individuals, families, groups, organizations, communities, and colleagues
- EP 2.1.4c Recognize and communicate their understanding of the importance of difference in shaping life experiences
- EP 2.1.7a Utilize conceptual frameworks to guide the processes of assessment, intervention, and evaluation
- EP 2.1.10a Substantively and affectively prepare for action with individuals, families, groups, organizations, and communities
- EP 2.1.10b Use empathy and other interpersonal skills
- EP 2.1.10d Collect, organize, and interpret client data
- EP 2.1.10e Assess client strengths and limitations

A. Brief Description

You will select and interview an individual while following an outline that indicates the information you need to solicit. The information reflects the types of information typically gathered by social workers in practice when doing a social history. Social histories reflect the important aspects of an individual's development and help social workers assess the nature of a client's problems.

B. Objectives

This exercise will enable you to:

1. Identify those aspects of human development that are important in shaping an individual's life situation and issues.
2. Recognize the complexity and necessity of assessment in social work practice.
3. Experience the process of interviewing and recognize the need to develop interviewing skills.

C. Procedure

1. Choose a person to interview. This could be a friend, a relative, or an acquaintance. Describe this assignment to the person, and ask the person for permission to do the interview. Feel free to show the person these guidelines or your proposed outline ahead of time. Make it clear that his or her real name will not be used and that the information will be kept confidential. Your instructor will provide additional information regarding how to conduct the interview.

    In practice, a social history involves "an in-depth description and assessment of the current and past client situation, often included in the case records and medical records of clients" (Barker, 2003, p. 404). The purpose is not to learn every intimate detail of the client's personal life but rather to gain a generalized understanding of what a client's life is like in addition to gaining more specific information related to the client's problem.

The Social History Outline developed for this assignment is not a complete social history but only portions of one. There are no sections that relate to problems or to recommendations. This assignment does not focus on a client's problem, because you have neither client nor problem to work with. However, this assignment is designed to give you a chance to interview someone, obtain developmental and social information, and summarize this information in an organized, informative manner.

2. One requirement of the assignment is to go to the library and do some related research on interviewing techniques. Look for information on what is involved in interviewing and how to do it. Summarize the research and information you reviewed and include it in the "Research Applications" section of the paper. Apply this research and information to your own interview where possible. For example, which techniques did you find useful or could you have used? How were they, or might they have been, helpful in your interview situation?

   Include a brief bibliography of all your references at the end of the paper.

3. Use the following outline when conducting the interview. Note that, at times, the outline includes specific questions you might want to ask.

   This is simply a guideline for you to use. In some cases you might have to ask more questions to get sufficient information. In other cases, the questions may not apply. In these cases, you should state that they don't apply. You should also make it clear when information is unavailable.

SOCIAL HISTORY OUTLINE

I. Basic Data

Client: (Legal name plus nickname) | Date of Birth:

Chronological Age: | Race:

Religion: | School and Grade:

Place of Employment: (if appropriate) | Address:

Telephone Number:

II. Individual Client Profile

A. Brief Physical Description of Client—Personality Picture

1. Describe the person's physical appearance (e.g., tall or short; color of hair). You might include information about dress, posture, and facial expressions.

2. Mention anything that's striking about the individual.

3. Describe your impression of the person's personality (e.g., outgoing; soft-spoken; nervous).

---

4. Mention specific behaviors, if appropriate, that describe exactly what you mean (e.g., "She seemed nervous, as she constantly fidgeted in her chair and rapped her knuckles on the desk"). This might include information about motor activity, unusual mannerisms, and the client's reactions to you, the interviewer.

5. Be brief, clear, and specific.

B. Developmental History Questions

1. Pregnancy

a. Was your mother's pregnancy normal; uneventful; problematic?

b. Describe any problems or unusual circumstances.

2. Delivery

a. Was the delivery normal; routine; difficult/problematic?

b. Identify difficulties, problems, or unusual circumstances.

c. Provide APGAR score, if available.

d. Type of delivery (e.g., vertex; breech).

e. Were you born at full term or prematurely? If premature, by how many months?

f. Where were you born?

3. Medical Problems

a. Did you experience any significant medical problems as a child that were out of the ordinary?

b. If so, please describe the problems and any treatment you might have received.

4. Developmental Milestones

a. Sat alone

b. Walked

c. First words

d. Toilet trained

5. Parental Care

a. Do you think that your parents found it difficult or easy to care for you as a child? Explain.

6. Social/Emotional Aspects

a. What were your peer relationships like during childhood?

b. How would you have described yourself as a child (e.g., outgoing; shy; bright)?

c. What types of play, activities, and hobbies did you participate in as a child?

d. How would you describe your childhood (e.g., happy; uneventful; turbulent)?

e. Were there any events that occurred during childhood that you feel significantly affected you? If so, describe the events and their effects.

7. Other

Is there any other information about your childhood that is important?

C. School History

1. Schools attended (names, dates, and locations)

2. Current school status (e.g., high school graduate; college sophomore)

3. Academic progress in schools (was school difficult for you?)

4. Attendance

5. Courses taken

6. Participation in school-related activities

7. Peer relationships (e.g., did you have friends in school? Did you feel liked by your classmates?)

8. Parental involvement with schools

9. Vocational history (special non-college job training)—type of training, dates, jobs, work record

D. Military Service

If applicable, describe the branch, rank, dates of service, duties, and type of discharge.

E. Employment History

1. Place, types, and dates of employment

2. Primary job responsibilities

3. Likes and dislikes about each job

4. Attendance record

5. Are you happy with your current employment? Explain.

F. Current Social/Emotional Elements

1. What are your social relationships like now? Would you say you are the type of person who has many friends or only a select few? Would you call yourself a lonely person?

2. Do you have any special relationships (e.g., girl/boyfriend; spouse)? If so, describe them. If married, elaborate under the following section, "Family History."

3. What are your major interests, activities, and hobbies? Describe them.

4. In summary, how would you describe your overall "fit" into a social context (e.g., generally popular; shy except with close friends)?

G. Self-Description

1. What do you like about yourself? What are your strengths?

2. What do you dislike about yourself?

3. Describe your current fears or worries.

4. What do you see as your personal accomplishments?

5. What is the most difficult thing you've accomplished? Why do you think this is so?

6. Describe the most painful event in your life.

7. What things would you like to change in your life and about yourself?

III. Family History

A. Family of Origin

1. Describe each family member in your family of origin. Include the following information:

   a. Relationship and name

   b. Date of birth and age

   c. Occupation

   d. Education

   e. Vocation and employment

   f. Current marital status

   g. Any major medical/psychological problems

   h. Brief description of physical appearance, personality, and how the person relates to other family members

2. Use the following format:

   Mother: (continue with above information)

   Father:

   Sister:

   Brother:

   Etc.

3. Family function

   a. What are marriage dates and current status (e.g., married; divorced)?

   b. Describe your parents' relationship.

   c. What types of family planning/birth control did your parents use?

   d. How does each of the other family members feel toward you?

   e. How do you get along with and relate to each of the other family members?

f. Are there any problems currently operating within the family? Were there any in the past? If so, explain.

g. Describe the socioeconomic (overall financial/living) conditions of your family now and during your childhood.

h. Did you have any special care situations during childhood (e.g., adoption; foster care)? If so, when did they occur and what were they like?

i. Did any significant stressful event occur in your family during your childhood? These might include deaths, domestic violence, drug/alcohol abuse, physical abuse, job loss, or other traumas. If so, explain.

j. How would you summarize the quality of your family life during your childhood?

k. Is there anything else about your family life during your childhood that you'd like to add?

4. Extended family

a. Briefly describe all people living or dead who are or were related to you. Include more detail for those relatives who are especially meaningful or significant to you.

b. Use the following format:

Maternal Grandmother:

Maternal Grandfather:

Paternal Aunt:

Etc.

B. <u>Current Family Relationships</u>

1. Marital status

a. Married, separated, single, widow/widower, divorced

b. Length of present marriage

c. How would you describe the quality of your present marriage (e.g., bad communication; enjoyable; full of conflict)?

d. Were you or your spouse married before?

e. If so, what were the dates, lengths of marriages, and reasons for terminating the marriage?

f. What are your socioeconomic (overall financial/living) conditions currently like?

2. Children

a. Names

b. Ages

c. Grade in school

d. Brief description of physical appearance and personality

e. How would you describe each child's behavior? How easy or difficult is each child to manage?

f. Relationships with peers and siblings.

IV. Summary Impression

In a few words, summarize the essentials of this history. If you had to describe this person and his/her life in a few words, what would you say?

V. Research Applications

This is not part of a regular social history. Please refer to Step 2 in the Procedures for instructions about completing this section.

3. Write a paper that summarizes the information you've gathered. The paper should be typewritten, double-spaced, and eight to twelve pages in length. Use an outline form for topic headings followed by a narrative presentation of information for each heading. Make sure each underlined topic heading is included in your paper.
4. The following provides an example of what your final social history might look like:

SOCIAL HISTORY EXAMPLE

I. Basic Data:

Client: Prudence Dill
Nickname: Pickles
Chronological Age: 18
Date of birth: August 31, 2004
Race: Caucasian
Religion: Roman Catholic
School: University of Wisconsin-Madison

Grade: Freshman
Place of Employment: Buster's Burger Palace
Address: 709 Main Street, Apt. 4, Nomansland, Wisconsin
Telephone: (414) 208-0009

II. Individual Client Profile:

A. Brief Physical-Personality Picture:

Prudence is a tall, thin, attractive young woman who has an energetic and responsive manner. She seemed interested in the interview and eager to provide information.

B. Gestation, Delivery, and Post-Natal Period:

Prudence is the third born in a family of five children. To her knowledge, her delivery was without any complications. She had no physical problems at birth or shortly thereafter. As far as she knows her parents had planned for her. Both parents had indicated they always wanted a large family. She felt they were very happy with her when she was born.

C. Development:

1. Medical:

Prudence was a consistently healthy child. She never had any serious diseases, allergies, accidents, or broken bones. She is up-to-date on her immunizations and has no sensory impairments. She avoids engaging in health hazards such as smoking, drugs, or unhealthy eating habits. However, she does engage in some moderate drinking. She lifts weights three times a week in addition to participating in other sports. These sports include wrestling and ice hockey. In summary, Prudence appears to be a healthy individual.

5. Following are some suggestions you might consider for improving the writing of professional reports such as social histories. They are in no particular order of importance or priority.

Use paragraphs to divide content into different topics/points/issues (avoid one-sentence paragraphs).

Avoid slang. Slang doesn't sound very professional. Don't use "guys." Use "young men" or "boys." Don't use "mom." Use "mother." Don't use "fizzled out." Use "didn't succeed" or something similar.

Avoid using words such as "always," "average," "perfect," or "all." (Who is "average"? Are you? What is perfect? Is someone "always" a happy person even after getting a D- on an exam for this course?)

Avoid sexist language. Use "Ms." instead of "Mrs." Use "woman" instead of "lady." Use "homemaker" or "woman who does not work outside of the home" instead of "housewife." Don't call adult women "girls."

Avoid using acronyms. Some people may not understand them. Spell the term out the first time and put the acronym in parentheses right after it. Thereafter, you can use just the acronym. For example, "The National Association of Social Workers (NASW) is the major professional organization for social work practitioners. NASW is a good organization to join."

Be as concise as possible. Look at a sentence and see if you could use fewer words. Consider dividing giant sentences into two or more smaller ones.

Distinguish between fact and your impression of what's going on. Ways to phrase your impressions include "My impression is . . .," "It appears that . . .," or "It seems that . . .".

Use apostrophes to indicate possession. For example, "Ronald's pet monkey is named Bonzo," or "Freddy's girlfriend jilted him when he was age 11."

It's shorter to state ages by saying, "Matilda, 108, . . ." instead of "Matilda was a woman who was 108 years old."

Spell correctly.

Avoid labeling people with terms like "low-life dirtball," "Mongoloid," "sleazy," or "abnormal."

Stress confidentiality. Don't use real names in this practice interview. Change some minor facts such as the specific community the person comes from if they are too revealing of her/his identity.

If you take notes during the interview, ask the client's permission first.

When you begin the interview, review its purpose and generally what you plan to do.

Competencies/Practice Behaviors Exercise 1.3
Writing Exercise Role-Play

Focus Competencies or Practice Behaviors:

- EP 2.1.3c Demonstrate effective oral and written communication in working with individuals, families, groups, organizations, communities, and colleagues

A. Brief Description

You will be asked to do a brief role-play in class to practice a portion of the social history. You will then practice a portion of the social history. You will then write up your findings and have a peer critique them.

B. Objectives

This exercise will enable you to:

1. Dramatize a portion of an interview through a role-play.
2. Evaluate a peer's and your own writing.
3. Employ suggestions to improve your writing.

C. Procedure

1. Your instructor will discuss Exercise 1.3, entitled Social History Assignment, and will specify a small portion of the assignment for use during a practice role-play.
2. Form pairs; one person will be the interviewer and one the interviewee. You will be given 10 minutes to collect and write down as much information as you can. The information should follow the portion of the social history outline that you've been instructed to address. This is to give you the chance to practice how to do your real social history interview. The interviewee should not give truthful information about her- or himself but should make up information to protect confidentiality.
3. After 10 minutes, exchange roles. The interviewer will now be the interviewee and vice versa. For the next 10 minutes, do the same role-play with your roles reversed.
4. You will be given another 10 minutes to write down the information you've gathered as if you were writing a real portion of a social history. Try to utilize the good writing suggestions you've been given.
5. Stop writing after 10 minutes have passed regardless of whether you've finished writing about all of the information. Exchange summaries with your role-play partner. Take another 5 minutes to critique each other's writing. Give constructive criticism regarding (a) writing style (grammar, spelling, clarity), and (b) accuracy of information, professional objectivity. Make suggestions to your partner, if you can, about how s/he might better present the information.
6. If there is time, your instructor may choose to critique some of the information summaries before the entire class. This may be done either by asking for volunteers, or by collecting all of the paragraphs anonymously and arbitrarily selecting one or two. The instructor will copy the information on the board and ask for constructive feedback from the class during the subsequent discussion.

REFERENCES: Barker, R. L. (2003). *The social work dictionary* (5th ed.). Washington, DC: NASW Press.

Competencies/Practice Behaviors Exercise 1.4
Introductory Ice-Breaker Role-Play

Focus Competencies or Practice Behaviors:

- EP 2.1.1b Practice personal reflection and self-correction to assure continual professional development
- EP 2.1.4b Gain sufficient self-awareness to eliminate the influence of personal biases and values in working with diverse groups

A. Brief Description

In this introductory exercise, you will introduce yourself and share something about yourself with other members of the class.

B. Objectives

You will:

1. Express some basic information about yourself.
2. Practice participating in class activities.
3. Examine some basic feelings about yourself.

C. Procedure

1. Arrange yourselves in a circle to allow for maximum eye contact among all group members.
2. On an 8" x 5" note card or a piece of scratch paper, draw six equal divisions and fill in the following information:

Upper Left-hand Corner: Write three adjectives that describe what you like about yourself.

Upper Right-hand Corner: Write three adjectives that describe what you dislike about yourself.

Left Center: State briefly why you are taking this course.

Right Center: State briefly what you expect to be doing five years from now, both personally and professionally.

Lower Left-hand Corner: State briefly what makes you angry.

Lower Right-hand Corner: State briefly what makes you happy.

You have approximately five minutes to jot down this information. You should self-disclose only the information you feel comfortable in sharing.

Chapter 1 Competencies/Practice Behaviors Exercises Assessment:

Name: ______________________________ **Date:** __________
Supervisor's Name: ____________________

Focus Competencies/Practice Behaviors:

- EP 2.1.1b Practice personal reflection and self-correction to assure continual professional development
- EP 2.1.3c Demonstrate effective oral and written communication in working with individuals, families, groups, organizations, communities, and colleagues
- EP 2.1.4b Gain sufficient self-awareness to eliminate the influence of personal biases and values in working with diverse groups
- EP 2.1.4c Recognize and communicate their understanding of the importance of difference in shaping life experiences
- EP 2.1.7a Utilize conceptual frameworks to guide the processes of assessment, intervention, and evaluation
- EP 2.1.10a Substantively and affectively prepare for action with individuals, families, groups, organizations, and communities
- EP 2.1.10b Use empathy and other interpersonal skills
- EP 2.1.10d Collect, organize, and interpret client data
- EP 2.1.10e Assess client strengths and limitations

Instructions:

A. Evaluate your work or your partner's work in the Focus Competencies/Practice Behaviors by completing the Competencies/Practice Behaviors Assessment form below

B. What other Competencies/Practice Behaviors did you use to complete these Exercises? Be sure to record them in your assessments

1.	I have attained this competency/practice behavior (in the range of 81 to 100%)
2.	I have largely attained this competency/practice behavior (in the range of 61 to 80%)
3.	I have partially attained this competency/practice behavior (in the range of 41 to 60%)
4.	I have made a little progress in attaining this competency/practice behavior (in the range of 21 to 40%)
5.	I have made almost no progress in attaining this competency/practice behavior (in the range of 0 to 20%)

EPAS 2008 Core Competencies & Core Practice Behaviors	Student Self Assessment						Evaluator Feedback
Student and Evaluator Assessment Scale and Comments	0	1	2	3	4	5	Agree/Disagree/Comments
EP 2.1.1 Identify as a Professional Social Worker and Conduct Oneself Accordingly:							
a. Advocate for client access to the services of social work							
b. Practice personal reflection and self-correction to assure continual professional development							
c. Attend to professional roles and boundaries							
d. Demonstrate professional demeanor in behavior, appearance, and communication							

e. Engage in career-long learning							
f. Use supervision and consultation							
EP 2.1.2 Apply Social Work Ethical Principles to Guide Professional Practice:							
a. Recognize and manage personal values in a way that allows professional values to guide practice							
b. Make ethical decisions by applying NASW Code of Ethics and, as applicable, of the IFSW/IASSW Ethics in Social Work, Statement of Principles							
c. Tolerate ambiguity in resolving ethical conflicts							
d. Apply strategies of ethical reasoning to arrive at principled decisions							
EP 2.1.3 Apply Critical Thinking to Inform and Communicate Professional Judgments:							
a. Distinguish, appraise, and integrate multiple sources of knowledge, including research-based knowledge and practice wisdom							
b. Analyze models of assessment, prevention, intervention, and evaluation							
c. Demonstrate effective oral and written communication in working with individuals, families, groups, organizations, communities, and colleagues							
EP 2.1.4 Engage Diversity and Difference in Practice:							
a. Recognize the extent to which a culture's structures and values may oppress, marginalize, alienate, or create or enhance privilege and power							
b. Gain sufficient self-awareness to eliminate the influence of personal biases and values in working with diverse groups							
c. Recognize and communicate their understanding of the importance of difference in shaping life experiences							
d. View themselves as learners and engage those with whom they work as informants							
EP 2.1.5 Advance Human Rights and Social and Economic Justice:							
a. Understand forms and mechanisms of oppression and discrimination							
b. Advocate for human rights and social and economic justice							
c. Engage in practices that advance social and economic justice							
EP 2.1.6 Engage in Research-Informed Practice and Practice-Informed Research:							
a. Use practice experience to inform scientific inquiry							
b. Use research evidence to inform practice							
EP 2.1.7 Apply Knowledge of Human Behavior and the Social Environment:							
a. Utilize conceptual frameworks to guide the processes of assessment, intervention, and evaluation							
b. Critique and apply knowledge to understand person and environment							

EP 2.1.8 Engage in Policy Practice to Advance Social and Economic Well-Being and to Deliver Effective Social Work Services:							
a. Analyze, formulate, and advocate for policies that advance social well-being							
b. Collaborate with colleagues and clients for effective policy action							
EP 2.1.9 Respond to Contexts that Shape Practice:							
a. Continuously discover, appraise, and attend to changing locales, populations, scientific and technological developments, and emerging societal trends to provide relevant services							
b. Provide leadership in promoting sustainable changes in service delivery and practice to improve the quality of social services							
EP 2.1.10 Engage, Assess, Intervene, and Evaluate with Individuals, Families, Groups, Organizations and Communities:							
a. Substantively and affectively prepare for action with individuals, families, groups, organizations, and communities							
b. Use empathy and other interpersonal skills							
c. Develop a mutually agreed-on focus of work and desired outcomes							
d. Collect, organize, and interpret client data							
e. Assess client strengths and limitations							
f. Develop mutually agreed-on intervention goals and objectives							
g. Select appropriate intervention strategies							
h. Initiate actions to achieve organizational goals							
i. Implement prevention interventions that enhance client capacities							
j. Help clients resolve problems							
k. Negotiate, mediate, and advocate for clients							
l. Facilitate transitions and endings							
m. Critically analyze, monitor, and evaluate interventions							

Chapter 2
Biological Development in Infancy and Childhood

Competencies/Practice Behaviors Exercise 2.1
The Abortion Decision Role-Play

Focus Competencies or Practice Behaviors:

- EP 2.1.1b Practice personal reflection and self-correction to assure continual professional development
- EP 2.1.2a Recognize and manage personal values in a way that allows professional values to guide practice
- EP 2.1.2c Tolerate ambiguity in resolving ethical conflicts
- EP 2.1.3c Demonstrate effective oral and written communication in working with individuals, families, groups, organizations, communities, and colleagues
- EP 2.1.10a Substantively and affectively prepare for action with individuals, families, groups, organizations, and communities
- EP 2.1.10b Use empathy and other interpersonal skills
- EP 2.1.10e Assess client strengths and limitations
- EP 2.1.10g Select appropriate intervention strategies
- EP 2.1.10j Help clients resolve problems

A. Brief Description

You will be provided with a vignette describing a case of unplanned pregnancy. You will determine your own personal opinions concerning abortion and then form small groups to discuss the various options available to the person described in the case. Finally, you will break into pairs and participate in a role-play that focuses on distinguishing between personal and professional values.

B. Objectives

You will:

1. Become aware of the alternatives available to a person in the situation of unplanned pregnancy.
2. Examine your own opinions toward the controversial issue of abortion.
3. Evaluate the distinction between personal and professional values.

C. Procedure

1. Read the following vignette:

> Marge is a 16-year-old high school sophomore who is two months pregnant. The father is Homer, a 17-year-old high school junior.
>
> Marge and Homer have been "going steady" for two years. They think they love each other. Marge is a cheerleader and Homer is a quarterback on the varsity football team. They're both involved in school activities and have never really thought much about the future. Marge hasn't told Homer yet. She's confused about what to do. She doesn't know how he'll react. Marge hasn't told her parents yet either. They're religious, and she's afraid they'll be terribly disappointed in her. What should she do?

2. After reading the vignette, imagine yourself in Marge's position. Determine what you would do according to your own value system and jot this decision down on a piece of scrap paper.
3. Break into groups of four to six persons. Discuss the various alternatives available to Marge and the possible positive and negative consequences of each alternative. Select one member of your group to write down each alternative and the positive and negative consequences of each alternative. DO NOT share your personal opinion about what Marge should do with the rest of your group.
4. You will have 10 to 15 minutes of small-group discussions. Then come together for a full-class discussion. Share what you discussed about the available alternatives. As you do so, each alternative, along with its potential positive and negative consequences, will be written on the board so that all may see them.
5. Now form pairs for a role-play. In each pair, one person plays Marge and the other a school social worker. The scene of the role-play is Marge talking to the social worker about her problem and what to do. The social worker should help Marge identify the various alternatives available to her and the consequences of each. The client should be helped to come to HER OWN DECISION. The role-play may continue for 15 to 20 minutes.
6. Come together once again for a full-class discussion. The following questions may be used to initiate discussion:
   a. How did it feel being in the place of the client or the school social worker?
   b. Did any of the people playing social workers have opinions concerning abortion that differed from the client's decision? If so, in what respect?
   c. How difficult was it to remain objective in view of having your own personal opinions?
   d. What did you learn about professional values from doing this exercise?
   e. What did you learn about what counseling might be like?

Competencies/Practice Behaviors Exercise 2.2
Abortion Related Ethical Dilemmas in Practice

Focus Competencies or Practice Behaviors:

- EP 2.1.2a Recognize and manage personal values in a way that allows professional values to guide practice
- EP 2.1.2b Make ethical decisions by applying standards of the National Association of Social Workers Code of Ethics and, as applicable, of the International Federation of Social Workers/International Association of Schools of Social Work Ethics in Social Work, Statement of Principles
- EP 2.1.2c Tolerate ambiguity in resolving ethical conflicts
- EP 2.1.2d Apply strategies of ethical reasoning to arrive at principled decisions

A. Brief Description

This exercise presents you with a variety of scenarios dramatizing ethical dilemmas concerning the abortion issue. In small groups you will discuss how a hierarchy of ethical principles might be applied, followed by a full-class discussion.

B. Objectives

You will:

1. Become aware of some of the ethical dilemmas that may be encountered in social work practice concerning the abortion issue.
2. Examine how a hierarchy of professional ethics can be applied.

C. Procedure

1. Review the following material (also presented in the text):

Picture yourself as a professional social worker in practice. What happens when your own personal values seriously conflict with those expressed by your client? A basic professional value clearly specified in the National Association of Social Workers (NASW) Code of Ethics is the right of clients to make their own decisions. Or, what happens when there are problems regardless of which solution you choose? What happens when, whatever you do, you are placed in the position of violating some professional ethic?

By definition, an ethical dilemma involves conflicting principles. When two or more ethical principles oppose each other, it's impossible to make a "correct" decision that satisfies both or all principles involved. There is no perfect solution.

For instance, if your 15-year-old client tells you that he plans to murder his mother, you are caught in an ethical dilemma. It is impossible to maintain confidentiality with your client (a basic social work professional value) and yet do all you can to protect his mother from harm.

A wide range of situations involving abortion can place workers in situations involving ethical dilemmas. Dolgoff, Loewenberg, and Harrington (2009) have formulated a hierarchy of ethical principles to provide a guide for making difficult decisions. When two ethical principles conflict, they suggest which principle should have priority. Principle 1 should take priority over principles 2 through 7, principle 2 should take priority over principles 3 through 7, and so on. The hierarchy can be helpful in working through difficult situations.

The hierarchy of ethical principles involves the following (p. 65-67):

Principle 1: **"Protection of life"** should be met first. This might include food, clothing, shelter, adequate income, and access to health services.

Principle 2: After basic survival needs, the principle of "**equality and inequality**" suggests that equal persons have the right to be treated equally and non-equal persons have the right to be treated differently if the inequality is relevant to the issue in question. It follows that people with lesser power or people in vulnerable positions may need special treatment.

Principle 3: Social workers should strive to make decisions that foster people's right to "**autonomy and freedom.**" People have the right to make decisions about how to behave and live their own lives as long as these decisions do not hamper other people's autonomy and freedom.

Principle 4: People should experience the "**least harm**" possible in any situation. This principle straightforwardly states that people have the basic right to be saved from injury. Furthermore, in the event of potential injury, social workers should choose the route causing the least injury possible, the least lasting harm or injury, and, finally, "the most easily reversible harm."

Principle 5: People have the right to pursue a good "**quality of life.**" Social workers should choose options that enhance the quality of life for individuals and communities.

Principle 6: People's "**privacy and confidentiality**" should be fostered and maintained. However, these are less important than the well-being of all.

Principle 7: Practice decisions should allow workers to maintain "**truthfulness and full disclosure.**" Social workers should be able to provide any information that they deem necessary in any particular situation. However, the truth should not be told for its own sake when it violates a client's confidentiality.

2. Break up into small groups of four to six persons. Eight scenarios depicting ethical dilemmas are presented below (the first provides an example of how to proceed). For each scenario, discuss how Dolgoff and his colleagues' hierarchy of ethical principles for decision making might be applied. Starting with principle 1 and continuing through principle 7, evaluate how the ethical principles can be involved in each dilemma. Remember, there are no easy or "perfect" answers.
3. Read the following situation and its subsequent discussion of ethical principles as an example of how to discuss the others.

SCENARIO A: A 16-year-old young woman is raped and impregnated by a 40-year-old man as she is walking home from school one night. Both she and her parents are horrified and plagued with worry. They come to you for help. The girl desperately wants an abortion.

APPLICATION OF ETHICAL PRINCIPLES TO SCENARIO A: Consider Principle 1, the need to protect life. If you *personally* adopt an antiabortion stance and feel that abortion is murder, what do you do? A professional social worker's personal values must be acknowledged yet put aside in professional situations. In this case, the young woman and her parents want her to have the abortion.

We then look at Principle 2, which calls for the nurturance of equality and the combating of inequality. According to this principle, people should be treated equally. In this case they should have equal access to services. A neighboring state, its border only 25 miles away, allows abortions for all women who want them within the first trimester. Is this fair? Is this ethical? Should you help the young woman and her parents seek an abortion in a state that has different rules? Or should you work actively in your own state to advocate for change so that abortion would be a legal alternative for clients such as this?

Now consider Principle 3, which stresses people's right to autonomy, independence, and freedom. The young woman has the right to make her own decision. Your state might legally allow abortions for all women seeking them, or it might restrict them to only those women who have been raped or sexually abused. Or your state might ban all abortions unless the life of the mother is critically endangered.

If an abortion is legal in your state for a teenager like this, you as a worker can help her get one. She has made her decision. It is her legal right. However, if your state does not allow her to have a legal abortion, you are confronted with another dilemma.

Another potential issue to explore with women experiencing unwanted pregnancy concerns a woman's spiritual beliefs. What are her beliefs about this situation and how do they affect not only her ultimate decision, but also the psychological results of that decision?

Principle 4 refers to choosing options that result in the least harm to those involved. What kind of harm or potential harm might each of the people involved suffer? How might you measure the severity of harm?

Principle 5 reflects the importance of maintaining an optimum quality of life. If this young woman is prevented from having an abortion, how might her future be affected? In what ways might she lose control over her life? How will her short-term and long-term quality of life be affected?

Does Principle 6, the right to privacy and confidentiality, concern this situation? It is your responsibility to maintain your client's confidentiality.

How does Principle 7 concerning truthfulness and full disclosure apply? Can you provide the young woman and her parents with information that will help them pursue their chosen alternative? Should you share with them your personal views about what should be done? Or should you strive to maintain professional objectivity?

This discussion raises questions and issues. Each case is unique. Circumstances and attitudes vary widely. It is a professional social worker's ethical responsibility to resolve dilemmas and help clients solve problems to the best of that worker's ability. Each client should be helped to identify alternatives, evaluate the pros and cons of each, and come to a final decision. There are no absolute answers or perfect solutions.

Abortion provides an especially difficult issue because of people's strong opinions either against abortion or in favor of free choice. For this specific issue, the National Association of Social Workers (NASW) has established policy statements to help provide direction (NASW, 2009). Relevant statements read:

"As social workers, we support the right of individuals to decide for themselves, without duress and according to their own personal beliefs and convictions, whether they want to become parents, how many children they are willing and able to nurture, the opportune time for them to have children, and with whom they may choose to parent. …To support self-determination, … reproductive health services, including abortion services, must be legally, economically, and geographically accessible to all who need them. … Denying people with low income access to the full range of contraceptive methods, abortion, and sterilization services, and the educational programs that explain them, perpetuate poverty and the dependence on welfare programs and support the status quo of class stratification. … NASW supports …

- A woman's right to obtain an abortion, performed according to accepted medical standards and in an environment free of harassment or threat for both patients and providers.

- Reproductive health services, including abortion services, that are confidential, available at a reasonable cost, and covered in public and private health insurance plans on a par with other kinds of health services (contraceptive equity).

- Improved access to the full range of reproductive health services, including abortion services, for groups currently underserved in the United States, including people with low income and those who rely on Medicaid[1] to pay for their health care" (NASW, 2009, p. 129).

[1] *Medicaid* is a public assistance program established in 1965 and funded by federal and state governments, that pays for medical and hospital services for eligible people, determined to be in need, who are unable to pay for these services themselves.

"The NASW Code of Ethics (NASW, 2008) states that 'social workers promote clients' socially responsible self-determination' (p. 5). Self-determination means that without government interference, people can make their own decisions about sexuality and reproduction. It requires working toward safe, legal, and accessible reproductive health care services, including abortion services, for everyone" (p. 147).

4. In a similar manner, discuss the following scenarios, one by one. Apply the hierarchy of ethical principles to each.

SCENARIO B: A 45-year-old grandmother becomes pregnant. She already has seven children. Her personal physician refused to prescribe birth control pills for her because of her age and other health reasons. Nor did he discuss other forms of birth control with her or offer her the alternative of sterilization. Physically, it would be hazardous for her to have any more children. She comes to you, distraught and crying. She doesn't know what to do.

SCENARIO C: A woman of 32 who has a severe cognitive disability becomes pregnant. She is not capable of taking care of herself independently. However, she is easy prey and has a history of numerous sexual encounters. Her genetic background indicates that there is a high probability that she would have a child with a cognitive disability. It is clear that she would be unable to care for any child herself.

SCENARIO D: A 19-year-old college student is six weeks pregnant. She's been going with her boyfriend for the past seven months. For the past three months they have been seeing only each other, but don't consider themselves "serious" as yet. She had been using a diaphragm and contraceptive cream, but they failed to protect her. She doesn't want a baby right now. However, she feels terribly guilty about getting pregnant.

SCENARIO E: A married 24-year-old woman is pregnant. She already has one child with genetic defects. She and her husband have been through genetic evaluation and counseling at a local university. The conclusion is that since both parents have significant genetic problems, the chances for a normal child are extremely unlikely. The couple was deciding on a sterilization procedure when she became pregnant.

SCENARIO F: A married 28-year-old medical technician has been unaware of being pregnant until now, the seventh week of gestation. Throughout her entire pregnancy she has been exposing herself to dangerous X-ray radiation. The possibility that her fetus has been damaged from the radiation is very high. She and her husband want children at some time, but they dread the thought of having a baby who has serious impairments.

SCENARIO G: Four months ago a married man of 42 had a vasectomy. His 41-year-old wife just found out she is five weeks pregnant. Some sperm apparently had still been evident in his semen. They already have three teenage children. They adamantly do not want any more.

SCENARIO H: A 14-year-old high school student is pregnant. It just happened one night when she was out drinking. She never really considered using contraception. She's shocked that she's pregnant and is having difficulty thinking about the future.

5. After approximately one-half hour, your instructor calls you back together to participate in a group discussion. Individuals have an opportunity to share either their own feelings or issues discussed in the small groups. Address the following questions:

   a. What ethical principles did you find to be the most useful for each case?
   b. For each case, what do you think should be done?
   c. To what extent was the ethical hierarchy helpful for thinking each scenario through?
   d. To what extent do you think that the ethical hierarchy would be helpful in addressing other ethical dilemmas encountered in social work practice?
   e. To what extent do you agree with the hierarchy of ethical principles?
   f. Which situations were the most difficult to address and why?

Competencies/Practice Behaviors Exercise 2.3
The Infertility Crisis

Focus Competencies or Practice Behaviors:

- EP 2.1.1b Practice personal reflection and self-correction to assure continual professional development
- EP 2.1.2a Recognize and manage personal values in a way that allows professional values to guide practice

A. Brief Description
Within a small group format, you will explore your own feelings about infertility and delineate the alternatives available to infertile couples.

B. Objectives
You will:
1. Become aware of the alternatives available to infertile couples and evaluate the consequences of each.
2. Identify your own feelings about infertility.
3. Recognize the need to employ empathy toward clients in this position.

C. Procedure
1. Complete the following statement:
   If I were infertile, I would ______________________________.
   Record your answer on a piece of scratch paper. You have a few minutes to think about and write down your feelings.
2. Form groups of four to six persons. Discuss the following questions within your group.
   a. What are the alternatives available to infertile couples and the respective advantages and disadvantages of each?
   b. How would you feel if you found that you were infertile?
   c. What feelings do you think infertile couples might experience?
   d. What types of information and support do you think would be most helpful for an infertile couple?

3. You will have 15 minutes of small-group discussion, then come together and summarize and discuss the groups' findings.

Competencies/Practice Behaviors Exercise 2.4
Developmental Assessment

Focus Competencies or Practice Behaviors:

- EP 2.1.3a Distinguish, appraise, and integrate multiple sources of knowledge, including research-based knowledge and practice wisdom
- EP 2.1.6b Use research evidence to inform practice
- EP 2.1.7b Critique and apply knowledge to understand person and environment
- EP 2.1.10a Substantively and affectively prepare for action with individuals, families, groups, organizations, and communities
- EP 2.1.10e Assess client strengths and limitations

A. Brief Description

The instructor will present a series of vignettes that profile children of various ages. You will discuss whether each child is normal or is experiencing developmental lags.

B. Objectives

You will:

1. Relate motor, play, adaptive, social, and language milestones that characterize various ages.
2. Apply this information to making assessment decisions.

C. Procedure

1. One at a time, you are provided with the following vignettes. After each vignette, evaluate the extent to which each child fits the "normal" developmental profile. Focus on whether the motor, play, adaptive, social, and language milestones are appropriate for the child's age level. What types of referrals might be appropriate for those children who display developmental lags in various areas?

a. Kenji, age 2 years, can walk well but still runs with an awkward gait. He likes to play with and push large objects such as wagons and walkers. He also likes to play alongside other children but is not able to play with them in a cooperative fashion. His vocabulary includes about twenty-five words, but he is not yet very adept at putting two to three words together in order to express an idea.

b. Chaniqwa, age 4 years, is very active physically. She enjoys running, skipping, jumping, and performing stunts. She can use the bathroom by herself. She has a substantial vocabulary, although she has a tendency to misuse words and use improper grammar.

c. Wyanet, age 1 year, is able to balance her head at a 90-degree angle. She can also lift her head when placed on her stomach in a prone position. She is not yet able to sit alone. She can recognize her bottle and her mother. Verbalizations include gurgling, babbling, and cooing.

d. Sheridan, age 5 years, can draw simple, although recognizable, pictures. Dominance of her left hand has become well established. She can readily dress and undress herself. She enjoys playing in groups of other children and can cooperate with them quite well. She has a vocabulary of about fifty words. She can use pronouns such as *I* and prepositions such as *on* and *above* appropriately. She can put two or three words together and use them appropriately, although she has difficulty formulating longer phrases and sentences.

e. Luis, age 18 months, can crawl well but is unable to stand by himself. He likes to scribble with crayons and build with blocks. However, it is difficult for him to place even three or four blocks on top of each other. He can say a few sounds, including *mama* and *dada,* but cannot yet understand the meaning of words.

REFERENCES

Dolgoff, R., Loewenberg, F. M., & Harrington, D. (2009). *Ethical decisions for social work practice* (8th ed.). Belmont, CA: Brooks/Cole.

National Association of Social Workers. (2008). *Code of ethics.* Washington, DC: Author.

National Association of Social Workers. (2009). *Social work speaks: National Association of Social Workers Policy Statements 2009-2012* (8th ed.). Washington, DC: Author.

Chapter 2 Competencies/Practice Behaviors Exercises Assessment:

Name: ______________________ **Date:** __________
Supervisor's Name: ______________________

Focus Competencies/Practice Behaviors:

- EP 2.1.1b Practice personal reflection and self-correction to assure continual professional development
- EP 2.1.2a Recognize and manage personal values in a way that allows professional values to guide practice
- EP 2.1.2b Make ethical decisions by applying standards of the National Association of Social Workers Code of Ethics and, as applicable, of the International Federation of Social Workers/International Association of Schools of Social Work Ethics in Social Work, Statement of Principles
- EP 2.1.2c Tolerate ambiguity in resolving ethical conflicts
- EP 2.1.2d Apply strategies of ethical reasoning to arrive at principled decisions
- EP 2.1.3a Distinguish, appraise, and integrate multiple sources of knowledge, including research-based knowledge and practice wisdom
- EP 2.1.3c Demonstrate effective oral and written communication in working with individuals, families, groups, organizations, communities, and colleagues
- EP 2.1.6b Use research evidence to inform practice
- EP 2.1.7b Critique and apply knowledge to understand person and environment
- EP 2.1.10a Substantively and affectively prepare for action with individuals, families, groups, organizations, and communities
- EP 2.1.10b Use empathy and other interpersonal skills
- EP 2.1.10e Assess client strengths and limitations
- EP 2.1.10g Select appropriate intervention strategies
- EP 2.1.10j Help clients resolve problems

Instructions:

A. Evaluate your work or your partner's work in the Focus Competencies/Practice Behaviors by completing the Competencies/Practice Behaviors Assessment form below

B. What other Competencies/Practice Behaviors did you use to complete these Exercises? Be sure to record them in your assessments

1.	I have attained this competency/practice behavior (in the range of 81 to 100%)
2.	I have largely attained this competency/practice behavior (in the range of 61 to 80%)
3.	I have partially attained this competency/practice behavior (in the range of 41 to 60%)
4.	I have made a little progress in attaining this competency/practice behavior (in the range of 21 to 40%)
5.	I have made almost no progress in attaining this competency/practice behavior (in the range of 0 to 20%)

EPAS 2008 Core Competencies & Core Practice Behaviors	Student Self Assessment						Evaluator Feedback
Student and Evaluator Assessment Scale and Comments	**0**	**1**	**2**	**3**	**4**	**5**	**Agree/Disagree/Comments**
EP 2.1.1 Identify as a Professional Social Worker and Conduct Oneself Accordingly:							
a. Advocate for client access to the services of social work							
b. Practice personal reflection and self-correction to assure continual professional development							
c. Attend to professional roles and boundaries							
d. Demonstrate professional demeanor in behavior, appearance, and communication							
e. Engage in career-long learning							
f. Use supervision and consultation							
EP 2.1.2 Apply Social Work Ethical Principles to Guide Professional Practice:							
a. Recognize and manage personal values in a way that allows professional values to guide practice							
b. Make ethical decisions by applying NASW Code of Ethics and, as applicable, of the IFSW/IASSW Ethics in Social Work, Statement of Principles							
c. Tolerate ambiguity in resolving ethical conflicts							
d. Apply strategies of ethical reasoning to arrive at principled decisions							
EP 2.1.3 Apply Critical Thinking to Inform and Communicate Professional Judgments:							
a. Distinguish, appraise, and integrate multiple sources of knowledge, including research-based knowledge and practice wisdom							
b. Analyze models of assessment, prevention, intervention, and evaluation							
c. Demonstrate effective oral and written communication in working with individuals, families, groups, organizations, communities, and colleagues							
EP 2.1.4 Engage Diversity and Difference in Practice:							
a. Recognize the extent to which a culture's structures and values may oppress, marginalize, alienate, or create or enhance privilege and power							
b. Gain sufficient self-awareness to eliminate the influence of personal biases and values in working with diverse groups							
c. Recognize and communicate their understanding of the importance of difference in shaping life experiences							
d. View themselves as learners and engage those with whom they work as informants							
EP 2.1.5 Advance Human Rights and Social and Economic Justice:							
a. Understand forms and mechanisms of oppression and discrimination							

b. Advocate for human rights and social and economic justice							
c. Engage in practices that advance social and economic justice							
EP 2.1.6 Engage in Research-Informed Practice and Practice-Informed Research:							
a. Use practice experience to inform scientific inquiry							
b. Use research evidence to inform practice							
EP 2.1.7 Apply Knowledge of Human Behavior and the Social Environment:							
a. Utilize conceptual frameworks to guide the processes of assessment, intervention, and evaluation							
b. Critique and apply knowledge to understand person and environment							
EP 2.1.8 Engage in Policy Practice to Advance Social and Economic Well-Being and to Deliver Effective Social Work Services:							
a. Analyze, formulate, and advocate for policies that advance social well-being							
b. Collaborate with colleagues and clients for effective policy action							
EP 2.1.9 Respond to Contexts that Shape Practice:							
a. Continuously discover, appraise, and attend to changing locales, populations, scientific and technological developments, and emerging societal trends to provide relevant services							
b. Provide leadership in promoting sustainable changes in service delivery and practice to improve the quality of social services							
EP 2.1.10 Engage, Assess, Intervene, and Evaluate with Individuals, Families, Groups, Organizations and Communities:							
a. Substantively and affectively prepare for action with individuals, families, groups, organizations, and communities							
b. Use empathy and other interpersonal skills							
c. Develop a mutually agreed-on focus of work and desired outcomes							
d. Collect, organize, and interpret client data							
e. Assess client strengths and limitations							
f. Develop mutually agreed-on intervention goals and objectives							
g. Select appropriate intervention strategies							
h. Initiate actions to achieve organizational goals							
i. Implement prevention interventions that enhance client capacities							
j. Help clients resolve problems							
k. Negotiate, mediate, and advocate for clients							
l. Facilitate transitions and endings							
m. Critically analyze, monitor, and evaluate interventions							

Chapter 3
Psychological Development in Infancy and Childhood

Competencies/Practice Behaviors Exercise 3.1
To See or Not to See

Focus Competencies or Practice Behaviors:

- EP 2.1.1b Practice personal reflection and self-correction to assure continual professional development
- EP 2.1.4a Recognize the extent to which a culture's structures and values may oppress, marginalize, alienate, or create or enhance privilege and power
- EP 2.1.4b Gain sufficient self-awareness to eliminate the influence of personal biases and values in working with diverse groups
- EP 2.1.4c Recognize and communicate their understanding of the importance of difference in shaping life experiences
- EP 2.1.10b Use empathy and other interpersonal skills

A. Brief Description

You will be asked to read an exercise designed to simulate some of the visual perceptual problems experienced by people with this type of learning disability. Discussion follows regarding the difficulty and frustration involved.

B. Objectives

You will:

1. Recognize some of the difficulties facing people with visual perceptual problems.
2. Examine your own feelings and frustration during such an experience.
3. Employ empathy toward people with learning disabilities that involve visual perceptual problems.

C. Procedure

1. Read the following from this manual (or on a handout):

INSTRUCTIONS: The wollofgni alanogies have been belevopeb to ehnance ruoy aditily to unberstanb adsrtatc nocpects. Fro aech hter aeret wo se patare tastements. The fristil lusrtates woh wot se patare nocpects ro ibae s rae rael teb to aech ohter. The seco nb pari rp ovibse an popro tuni yt for yuo to lerate hte adsr tatc nocpect to anohter nocgif uratoin of wrobs. The byabs rae srtutcureb to rpe se nt vraoiusl evles ofb fificulyt. It si ver yim pr

o

t

n

a

t ht at yuobo not llif ni nay fo hte dl ank ps acse utnil yuo rae ins rtutceb to boso. In hte e vetn htat yuow riet an yhtgni no htis hse et defore degni insrtutceb to boso, uyo lliw imme biateyl cerie vea liafgni grabe for htis cuo rse:

1. Birds have xxxxx; people have ——.
2. xxxxx are mammals; ostriches are ——.
3. A yard has feet; a —— has xxxxx.
4. A banana is xxxxx; an apple is ——.
5. Tigers are xxxxx; pets are ——.
6. xxxxx is cold; —— is hot.
7. A volleyball is ——; a pickle is xxxxx.
8. —— are brave; xxxxx are docile.
9. Plants have xxxxx; trees have ——.
10. Doctors have patients; xxxxx have ——.

2. This activity simulates several aspects of what a person with a learning disability involving a visual perceptual problem may experience. Read the instructions and follow them very carefully. You will have 5 to 10 minutes.
3. Discuss what it is like to be a person with a learning disability. The following questions may be asked:
   a. How did it feel to attempt following the instructions?
   b. What adjectives might you use to describe your feelings during the activity?
   c. How might a person react if placed in a similar situation in real life?
   d. How might you react if you were placed in a situation where everyone else appears to know what to do, but you don't?
   e. What might be done to help a person in such a situation?
4. After voicing your feelings and opinions, read the following from this manual (or from a handout):

INSTRUCTIONS: The following analogies have been developed to enhance your ability to understand abstract concepts. For each there are two separate statements. The first illustrates how two separate concepts or ideas are related to each other. The second pair provides an opportunity for you to relate the abstract concept to another configuration of words. The dyads are structured to present various levels of difficulty. It is very important that you do not fill in any of the blank spaces until you are instructed to do so. In the event that you write anything on this sheet before being instructed to do so, you will immediately receive a failing grade for this course.

1. Birds have beaks; people have ——.
2. Rhinoceroses are mammals; ostriches are ——.
3. A yard has feet; a —— has inches.
4. A banana is yellow; an apple is ——.
5. Tigers are wild; pets are ——.
6. Winter is cold; —— is hot.

7. A volleyball is ——; a pickle is oblong.
8. —— are brave; sheep are docile.
9. Plants have stems; trees have ——.
10. Doctors have patients; social workers have ——.

5. After you have read these instructions, discussion may be continued by asking the following questions:
   a. How have your perceptions changed regarding how difficult the material is for you to understand?
   b. What types of information were lacking? What became unclear?
   c. How many of you began completing the first analogy sheet, even though the instructions told you not to?
   d. What might it feel like to fail at an assignment considered fairly simple by your peers?

Competencies/Practice Behaviors Exercise 3.2
I Don't Hear Anything, Do You?

Focus Competencies or Practice Behaviors:

- EP 2.1.1b Practice personal reflection and self-correction to assure continual professional development
- EP 2.1.4a Recognize the extent to which a culture's structures and values may oppress, marginalize, alienate, or create or enhance privilege and power
- EP 2.1.4b Gain sufficient self-awareness to eliminate the influence of personal biases and values in working with diverse groups
- EP 2.1.4c Recognize and communicate their understanding of the importance of difference in shaping life experiences
- EP 2.1.10b Use empathy and other interpersonal skills

A. Brief Description

You will be given verbal instructions to perform a complicated task under distracting conditions. After you try to do so, discuss the difficulties and frustrations you experienced.

B. Objectives

You will:

1. Recognize some of the difficulties facing people with auditory perceptual problems.
2. Examine your own feelings and frustration during such an experience.
3. Employ empathy toward people with learning disabilities that involve auditory perceptual problems.

C. Procedure

1. An audiotape of some type of muffled or distracting noise is prepared. The tape may be of the entire class holding small-group discussions, freeway traffic, or jazz music.
2. You are asked to complete a task by following verbal instructions. Meanwhile, the instructor plays the prerecorded tape at a relatively loud volume.
3. Have a pen or pencil ready. Do not begin work until the instructions have been completely read.

4. You have a few minutes to struggle with the exercise. The instructions will not be repeated. This activity simulates what a person with a learning disability involving an auditory perceptual problem may experience.
   a. How did it feel to attempt to follow the instructions?
   b. What adjectives might you use to describe your feelings during the activity?
   c. To what extent do you feel that the instructions and the learning situation were fair?
   d. What exactly might have made you confused during this exercise?
   e. How might a person with a learning disability feel in a similar situation in real life where all of his or her peers are capable of performing the task?

Competencies/Practice Behaviors Exercise 3.3
Developing a Positive Self-Concept

Focus Competencies or Practice Behaviors:

- EP 2.1.1b Practice personal reflection and self-correction to assure continual professional development
- EP 2.1.4c Recognize and communicate their understanding of the importance of difference in shaping life experiences
- EP 2.1.10b Use empathy and other interpersonal skills

A. Brief description

You will explore your self-concepts and then relate your findings to the general idea of a positive self-concept. Small group discussions follow.

B. Objectives

You will:

1. Identify those aspects of your own circumstances and personality that act to enhance or degrade your self-concept.
2. Relate this information to how others might develop and maintain their self-concepts.
3. Examine possible strategies for strengthening your self-concept.

C. Procedure

1. Review the material in the text concerning self-concept and self-esteem. Jot down your answers to the following questions:
   a. What things (that people tell you; that you achieve; that you like about yourself) make you feel good about yourself?
   b. What things make you feel bad about yourself?

   Take 5 to 10 minutes to think and write down your ideas.
2. Break into groups of four to six persons. Discuss the following questions:
   a. What types of things can be done to enhance a person's self-concept?
   b. What types of things act to harm a person's self-concept?
3. After 10 to 15 minutes, the small-group discussions will end. Designate someone to share the findings of your group with the class. Have another person record the main points on the board so that everyone can focus on them. Be specific.
4. Summarize the findings of the entire group. Focus on both similarities and differences concerning how self-concepts are maintained. Relate findings to social work practice by discussing how social workers might act to enhance the self-concepts of clients. Examine what types of things discourage clients and harm their self-concepts.

Competencies/Practice Behaviors Exercise 3.4
Who's the Smartest of Them All?

Focus Competencies or Practice Behaviors:

- EP 2.1.1b Practice personal reflection and self-correction to assure continual professional development
- EP 2.1.4a Recognize the extent to which a culture's structures and values may oppress, marginalize, alienate, or create or enhance privilege and power
- EP 2.1.4b Gain sufficient self-awareness to eliminate the influence of personal biases and values in working with diverse groups
- EP 2.1.4c Recognize and communicate their understanding of the importance of difference in shaping life experiences
- EP 2.1.10b Use empathy and other interpersonal skills

A. Brief description

You will be given questions concerning the differences and similarities among persons with varying levels of intelligence. Discussion will follow.

B. Objectives

You will:

1. Describe your perceptions of the effects of a person's intelligence on his or her behavior and the interaction between intelligence and personality.
2. Examine preconceived notions and stereotypes concerning persons of various levels of intelligence.
3. Recognize basic similarities and differences between people based on intellectual ability.

C. Procedure

1. The following three incomplete statements will be written on the board:
   a. People who have intellectual disabilities (formerly referred to as mental retardation) are:
   b. People with normal intelligence are:
   c. People with very high (far above normal) levels of intelligence are:
2. Break into groups of four to six. Discuss the feelings you think many people might have about persons of various levels of intelligence. Discuss not only your opinion but also stereotypes you think are frequently held. Record your findings. You will have 10 to 15 minutes for the small-group discussions.
3. Share your findings and record them on the board.
4. Continue with a discussion involving the entire class. Use the following questions to initiate this discussion:
   a. What major differences exist concerning the ideas about people of different levels of intelligence?
   b. How are people of all levels of intelligence thought to be similar?
   c. How do the following concepts relate to varying levels of ability:
      1) Emotional needs
      2) Intimate relationship need
      3) Self-concept
      4) Structure and supervision
      5) Work
      6) Right of free choice

d. How should people with very high levels of intelligence be treated? Should they be given more leadership responsibility? How do they interact with people of average intelligence?

e. What areas of life are most affected by levels of intelligence (e.g., family relationships, relationships with significant others, work, social life)?

f. From a social work perspective, how should people of different levels of intelligence be treated?

Competencies/Practice Behaviors Exercise 3.5
Everyday People Role-Play

Focus Competencies or Practice Behaviors:

- EP 2.1.1b Practice personal reflection and self-correction to assure continual professional development
- EP 2.1.4a Recognize the extent to which a culture's structures and values may oppress, marginalize, alienate, or create or enhance privilege and power
- EP 2.1.4b Gain sufficient self-awareness to eliminate the influence of personal biases and values in working with diverse groups
- EP 2.1.4c Recognize and communicate their understanding of the importance of difference in shaping life experiences
- EP 2.1.10b Use empathy and other interpersonal skills

A. Brief description

After reading about a child who has an IQ that is significantly below average attempting to interact with children of normal intelligence, you will be asked to discuss the alternatives.

B. Objectives

You will:

1. Recognize some of the effects of intellectual disability on an individual's self-concept and social interaction.
2. Examine alternatives for enhancing the social situation of a person who has such an intellectual disability.
3. Propose strategies for helping to integrate such an individual into a normal social setting.

C. Procedure

1. Bring this manual to class so that you might have the following material available:

SITUATION:

Mike, age 7, has been diagnosed as having a mild intellectual disability. He is a quiet, pleasant child who has difficulty keeping up with peers in schoolwork and in play/sport activities. He and his parents have moved into a new neighborhood filled with children of various ages.

QUESTIONS:

a. How do you think Mike might feel about himself in relationship to his peers?

b. How might the following people help to integrate Mike into the neighborhood:

1) Mike's parents

2) Neighbors

3) Other children
4) The school
5) Mike himself

2. Break into groups of four to six. After the situation is read aloud, discuss the subsequent questions. You will have 15 minutes for discussion.
3. A representative from each group summarizes what his or her group talked about. Then the class discusses the small groups' findings.
4. Summarize the conclusions of the entire group.

Chapter 3 Competencies/Practice Behaviors Exercises Assessment:

Name: ______________________________ **Date:** ____________
Supervisor's Name: ______________________________

Focus Competencies/Practice Behaviors:

- EP 2.1.1b Practice personal reflection and self-correction to assure continual professional development
- EP 2.1.4a Recognize the extent to which a culture's structures and values may oppress, marginalize, alienate, or create or enhance privilege and power
- EP 2.1.4b Gain sufficient self-awareness to eliminate the influence of personal biases and values in working with diverse groups
- EP 2.1.4c Recognize and communicate their understanding of the importance of difference in shaping life experiences
- EP 2.1.10b Use empathy and other interpersonal skills

Instructions:

A. Evaluate your work or your partner's work in the Focus Competencies/Practice Behaviors by completing the Competencies/Practice Behaviors Assessment form below

B. What other Competencies/Practice Behaviors did you use to complete these Exercises? Be sure to record them in your assessments

1.	I have attained this competency/practice behavior (in the range of 81 to 100%)
2.	I have largely attained this competency/practice behavior (in the range of 61 to 80%)
3.	I have partially attained this competency/practice behavior (in the range of 41 to 60%)
4.	I have made a little progress in attaining this competency/practice behavior (in the range of 21 to 40%)
5.	I have made almost no progress in attaining this competency/practice behavior (in the range of 0 to 20%)

EPAS 2008 Core Competencies & Core Practice Behaviors	Student Self Assessment						Evaluator Feedback
Student and Evaluator Assessment Scale and Comments	**0**	**1**	**2**	**3**	**4**	**5**	**Agree/Disagree/Comments**
EP 2.1.1 Identify as a Professional Social Worker and Conduct Oneself Accordingly:							
a. Advocate for client access to the services of social work							
b. Practice personal reflection and self-correction to assure continual professional development							
c. Attend to professional roles and boundaries							
d. Demonstrate professional demeanor in behavior, appearance, and communication							
e. Engage in career-long learning							
f. Use supervision and consultation							

EP 2.1.2 Apply Social Work Ethical Principles to Guide Professional Practice:							
a. Recognize and manage personal values in a way that allows professional values to guide practice							
b. Make ethical decisions by applying NASW Code of Ethics and, as applicable, of the IFSW/IASSW Ethics in Social Work, Statement of Principles							
c. Tolerate ambiguity in resolving ethical conflicts							
d. Apply strategies of ethical reasoning to arrive at principled decisions							
EP 2.1.3 Apply Critical Thinking to Inform and Communicate Professional Judgments:							
a. Distinguish, appraise, and integrate multiple sources of knowledge, including research-based knowledge and practice wisdom							
b. Analyze models of assessment, prevention, intervention, and evaluation							
c. Demonstrate effective oral and written communication in working with individuals, families, groups, organizations, communities, and colleagues							
EP 2.1.4 Engage Diversity and Difference in Practice:							
a. Recognize the extent to which a culture's structures and values may oppress, marginalize, alienate, or create or enhance privilege and power							
b. Gain sufficient self-awareness to eliminate the influence of personal biases and values in working with diverse groups							
c. Recognize and communicate their understanding of the importance of difference in shaping life experiences							
d. View themselves as learners and engage those with whom they work as informants							
EP 2.1.5 Advance Human Rights and Social and Economic Justice:							
a. Understand forms and mechanisms of oppression and discrimination							
b. Advocate for human rights and social and economic justice							
c. Engage in practices that advance social and economic justicep							
EP 2.1.6 Engage in Research-Informed Practice and Practice-Informed Research:							
a. Use practice experience to inform scientific inquiry							
b. Use research evidence to inform practice							

EP 2.1.7 Apply Knowledge of Human Behavior and the Social Environment:							
a. Utilize conceptual frameworks to guide the processes of assessment, intervention, and evaluation							
b. Critique and apply knowledge to understand person and environment							
EP 2.1.8 Engage in Policy Practice to Advance Social and Economic Well-Being and to Deliver Effective Social Work Services:							
a. Analyze, formulate, and advocate for policies that advance social well-being							
b. Collaborate with colleagues and clients for effective policy action							
EP 2.1.9 Respond to Contexts that Shape Practice:							
a. Continuously discover, appraise, and attend to changing locales, populations, scientific and technological developments, and emerging societal trends to provide relevant services							
b. Provide leadership in promoting sustainable changes in service delivery and practice to improve the quality of social services							
EP 2.1.10 Engage, Assess, Intervene, and Evaluate with Individuals, Families, Groups, Organizations and Communities:							
a. Substantively and affectively prepare for action with individuals, families, groups, organizations, and communities							
b. Use empathy and other interpersonal skills							
c. Develop a mutually agreed-on focus of work and desired outcomes							
d. Collect, organize, and interpret client data							
e. Assess client strengths and limitations							
f. Develop mutually agreed-on intervention goals and objectives							
g. Select appropriate intervention strategies							
h. Initiate actions to achieve organizational goals							
i. Implement prevention interventions that enhance client capacities							
j. Help clients resolve problems							
k. Negotiate, mediate, and advocate for clients							
l. Facilitate transitions and endings							
m. Critically analyze, monitor, and evaluate interventions							

Chapter 4
Social Development in Infancy and Childhood

Competencies/Practice Behaviors Exercise 4.1
The Family System Role-Play

Focus Competencies or Practice Behaviors:

- EP 2.1.7a Utilize conceptual frameworks to guide the processes of assessment, intervention, and evaluation
- EP 2.1.7b Critique and apply knowledge to understand person and environment

A. Brief description

You are presented with a description of a family and its members, followed by a series of situations occurring within the family. Discussion focuses on the direct application of systems concepts to this family and its situations.

B. Objectives

You will:

1. Examine the meanings of various systems theory concepts.
2. Apply these concepts to a series of concrete family life situations.

C. Procedure

1. After reviewing the systems theory concepts, join other students in a circle. This allows maximum observation of the activity.
2. The instructor describes the following family configuration:

WARD: Ward, age 41, is the husband and father. He can generally be described as calm and level-headed. He makes most of the family's decisions. Professionally, he's an accountant, earning an upper-middle-class income.

JUNE: June, age 35, is the wife and mother of the family. She can generally be described as pleasant, attractive, and warm. Although she is bright, she sometimes has difficulty asserting herself. She usually defers to Ward's opinions and decisions. She does not work outside the home.

WALTER: Walter is a pleasant, generally cooperative 16-year-old son. He has numerous friends, maintains a B+ grade average in school, and is interested in sports, especially football. He also loves cars and works on old wrecks whenever he has a chance in his free time.

BEVERLY: Beverly is 8 years old, and in third grade. She can generally be described as "cute." Although she is usually pleasant and cooperative, she has a tendency to get into minor trouble.

3. The instructor asks for volunteers to play each of the family members. The roles are written on 5" x 8" notecards and given to each role-player. The family members sit together inside the class circle. The role-players are given a series of situations. Each is

asked to respond as if he or she really was that family member. Role-players can add any additional details they wish about the family member.

4. The instructor presents the following situations to the family members:

   a. Ward loses his job. The family faces a financial crisis.
   b. The school principal calls and reports that Beverly was caught smoking in the school restroom.
   c. Walter tells the family that he wants to drop out of school to earn some money. He says he has a great offer to work at the local garage as a mechanic earning $7.50 an hour.
   d. June tells Ward that she's having an affair with the mailman.

5. Each family member tells how he or she feels about the situation and describes how the situation might affect the family.
6. After receiving feedback from the individual role-players, discuss the situations using systems theory concepts. Relate each systems theory term to the dynamics that might be occurring in the family. For example, any of the situations might upset the family's homeostasis. Other examples include how June's affair might affect the parental subsystem and how Ward's losing his job affects the amount of input (in this case, financial input) into the family.

Competencies/Practice Behaviors Exercise 4.2
Behavioral Description

Focus Competencies or Practice Behaviors:

- EP 2.1.3c Demonstrate effective oral and written communication in working with individuals, families, groups, organizations, communities, and colleagues
- EP 2.1.10a Substantively and affectively prepare for action with individuals, families, groups, organizations, and communities

A. Brief description

You will be asked to select, describe, observe, and determine the frequency of a behavior manifested by someone else in the room over a designated period of time. Discussion will focus on the importance of specificity in describing behavior.

B. Objectives

You will:

1. Describe a behavior in specific, measurable terms.
2. Examine the difficulty involved in behavioral definition.

C. Procedure

1. Arrange yourselves in a circle to allow for optimum observation of other students' behavior.
2. Take a few moments and select a specific behavior manifested by a particular individual in the room. Examples of such behaviors include blinking eyes, tapping feet, nodding heads, yawning, or swinging feet.
3. Describe your chosen behavior in writing.

4. You will have three minutes to count the number of times the specific behavior occurs. You will be told when to begin and when to stop your counting. Upon completion of your observation, write down the frequency of the behavior.
5. Discuss the specific behaviors selected. What difficulties did you encounter in attempting to complete this task? Select particular behaviors and illustrate how an arbitrary decision is sometimes involved in deciding whether a behavior did or did not occur. For example, how far must one's head move before it is considered a head turn? How distinctly must an eyelid flutter before the movement is considered to be a blink? Relate this task to problems of description and of monitoring child-behavior management. Emphasize the importance of behavioral specificity in order to measure improvements in behavior and to enhance accountability.

Competencies/Practice Behaviors Exercise 4.3
What's Wrong With the Program?

Focus Competencies or Practice Behaviors:

- EP 2.1.7a Utilize conceptual frameworks to guide the processes of assessment, intervention, and evaluation
- EP 2.1.7b Critique and apply knowledge to understand person and environment
- EP 2.1.10a Substantively and affectively prepare for action with individuals, families, groups, organizations, and communities
- EP 2.1.10d Collect, organize, and interpret client data
- EP 2.1.10e Assess client strengths and limitations
- EP 2.1.10g Select appropriate intervention strategies

A. Brief description
Several behavioral programs for children are described; you are to evaluate their potential effectiveness.

B. Objectives
You will:
1. Recognize potential problems in attempting to control behavior.
2. Assess the potential effectiveness of various behavioral techniques.
3. Propose effective alternative child-behavior management techniques.

C. Procedure
1. Several child-behavior management situations are described on small slips of paper, which are placed in an envelope. The situations may include, but are not limited to, the following:

a. Virgil, age 6, wets his pants an average of eight times a day. His mother decides to try to stop this behavior. She tells him that if he doesn't wet his pants the whole day he can have his dessert after dinner.
b. Koko's father is disgusted with Koko's childish behavior. Koko is 9 years old. He says that he will give her a nickel every time she acts her age.
c. Ahmed, age 11, is a sloppy eater. His mother states that if he doesn't change his eating habits, he'll have to go without supper.

d. Susie, age 7, teases her sister Karen, age 3. Susie takes Karen's Barbie doll and holds it high above her head so Karen can't reach it. As a result, Karen cries and screams. Their father decides this behavior has to stop. He tells Susie that if she doesn't stop it, he'll take her own favorite doll and give it to Karen.

e. Shirley, age 8, likes to jump off the tool shed into a big bale of hay. Her mother thinks this is much too dangerous and wants her to stop it. Her mother can usually see Shirley start climbing on the tool-shed roof from the kitchen window. Every time Shirley's mother sees Shirley climbing, she runs out of the house, grabs Shirley by the hand, pulls her into the house, and pleads with her to stop that climbing or she'll kill herself.

f. Rick, age 10, likes to annoy his brother Kevin, age 6. Rick does this by shooting an air gun at Kevin. Even though the air gun just shoots air, it makes a loud noise, and sometimes Rick aims it right into Kevin's ear. Their parents want this to stop, so they ignore the behavior, hoping that it will go away.

2. After reviewing the learning theory concepts and applications presented in the text, you will critique the behavioral situations. A volunteer draws one of the slips from the envelope, comments on the pros and cons of the program, and makes suggestions for improving it. After the student has a chance to comment, the rest of the class has an opportunity to evaluate the adequacy of the behavioral program.
3. The envelope is handed to the next student. This person follows the same procedure as the first, and then the discussion is again resumed by the entire class.
4. Repeat this procedure as frequently as time, numbers of situations, and interest allow.

Chapter 4 Competencies/Practice Behaviors Exercises Assessment:

Name: ______________________________ **Date:** __________
Supervisor's Name: ______________________________

Focus Competencies/Practice Behaviors:

- EP 2.1.3c Demonstrate effective oral and written communication in working with individuals, families, groups, organizations, communities, and colleagues
- EP 2.1.7a Utilize conceptual frameworks to guide the processes of assessment, intervention, and evaluation
- EP 2.1.7b Critique and apply knowledge to understand person and environment
- EP 2.1.10a Substantively and affectively prepare for action with individuals, families, groups, organizations, and communities
- EP 2.1.10d Collect, organize, and interpret client data
- EP 2.1.10e Assess client strengths and limitations
- EP 2.1.10g Select appropriate intervention strategies

Instructions:

A. Evaluate your work or your partner's work in the Focus Competencies/Practice Behaviors by completing the Competencies/Practice Behaviors Assessment form below

B. What other Competencies/Practice Behaviors did you use to complete these Exercises? Be sure to record them in your assessments

1.	I have attained this competency/practice behavior (in the range of 81 to 100%)
2.	I have largely attained this competency/practice behavior (in the range of 61 to 80%)
3.	I have partially attained this competency/practice behavior (in the range of 41 to 60%)
4.	I have made a little progress in attaining this competency/practice behavior (in the range of 21 to 40%)
5.	I have made almost no progress in attaining this competency/practice behavior (in the range of 0 to 20%)

EPAS 2008 Core Competencies & Core Practice Behaviors	**Student Self Assessment**						**Evaluator Feedback**
Student and Evaluator Assessment Scale and Comments	**0**	**1**	**2**	**3**	**4**	**5**	**Agree/Disagree/Comments**
EP 2.1.1 Identify as a Professional Social Worker and Conduct Oneself Accordingly:							
a. Advocate for client access to the services of social work							
b. Practice personal reflection and self-correction to assure continual professional development							
c. Attend to professional roles and boundaries							
d. Demonstrate professional demeanor in behavior, appearance, and communication							
e. Engage in career-long learning							
f. Use supervision and consultation							

EP 2.1.2 Apply Social Work Ethical Principles to Guide Professional Practice:							
a. Recognize and manage personal values in a way that allows professional values to guide practice							
b. Make ethical decisions by applying NASW Code of Ethics and, as applicable, of the IFSW/IASSW Ethics in Social Work, Statement of Principles							
c. Tolerate ambiguity in resolving ethical conflicts							
d. Apply strategies of ethical reasoning to arrive at principled decisions							
EP 2.1.3 Apply Critical Thinking to Inform and Communicate Professional Judgments:							
a. Distinguish, appraise, and integrate multiple sources of knowledge, including research-based knowledge and practice wisdom							
b. Analyze models of assessment, prevention, intervention, and evaluation							
c. Demonstrate effective oral and written communication in working with individuals, families, groups, organizations, communities, and colleagues							
EP 2.1.4 Engage Diversity and Difference in Practice:							
a. Recognize the extent to which a culture's structures and values may oppress, marginalize, alienate, or create or enhance privilege and power							
b. Gain sufficient self-awareness to eliminate the influence of personal biases and values in working with diverse groups							
c. Recognize and communicate their understanding of the importance of difference in shaping life experiences							
d. View themselves as learners and engage those with whom they work as informants							
EP 2.1.5 Advance Human Rights and Social and Economic Justice:							
a. Understand forms and mechanisms of oppression and discrimination							
b. Advocate for human rights and social and economic justice							
c. Engage in practices that advance social and economic justice							
EP 2.1.6 Engage in Research-Informed Practice and Practice-Informed Research:							
a. Use practice experience to inform scientific inquiry							
b. Use research evidence to inform practice							

EP 2.1.7 Apply Knowledge of Human Behavior and the Social Environment:						
a. Utilize conceptual frameworks to guide the processes of assessment, intervention, and evaluation						
b. Critique and apply knowledge to understand person and environment						
EP 2.1.8 Engage in Policy Practice to Advance Social and Economic Well-Being and to Deliver Effective Social Work Services:						
a. Analyze, formulate, and advocate for policies that advance social well-being						
b. Collaborate with colleagues and clients for effective policy action						
EP 2.1.9 Respond to Contexts that Shape Practice:						
a. Continuously discover, appraise, and attend to changing locales, populations, scientific and technological developments, and emerging societal trends to provide relevant services						
b. Provide leadership in promoting sustainable changes in service delivery and practice to improve the quality of social services						
EP 2.1.10 Engage, Assess, Intervene, and Evaluate with Individuals, Families, Groups, Organizations and Communities:						
a. Substantively and affectively prepare for action with individuals, families, groups, organizations, and communities						
b. Use empathy and other interpersonal skills						
c. Develop a mutually agreed-on focus of work and desired outcomes						
d. Collect, organize, and interpret client data						
e. Assess client strengths and limitations						
f. Develop mutually agreed-on intervention goals and objectives						
g. Select appropriate intervention strategies						
h. Initiate actions to achieve organizational goals						
i. Implement prevention interventions that enhance client capacities						
j. Help clients resolve problems						
k. Negotiate, mediate, and advocate for clients						
l. Facilitate transitions and endings						
m. Critically analyze, monitor, and evaluate interventions						

Chapter 5
Ethnocentrism and Racism

Competencies/Practice Behaviors Exercise 5.1
Stereotyping

Focus Competencies or Practice Behaviors:

- EP 2.1.1b Practice personal reflection and self-correction to assure continual professional development
- EP 2.1.4a Recognize the extent to which a culture's structures and values may oppress, marginalize, alienate, or create or enhance privilege and power
- EP 2.1.4b Gain sufficient self-awareness to eliminate the influence of personal biases and values in working with diverse groups
- EP 2.1.5a Understand forms and mechanisms of oppression and discrimination

A. Brief description

Some vignettes will be read, and you will be asked to identify the racial or ethnic groups described in the vignettes.

B. Objectives

You will:

1. Become aware that you, like everyone else, hold stereotypes about racial and ethnic groups.

C. Procedures

1. The instructor begins by reading to you, or asking you to read, the vignettes that follow. Write down the name(s) of the racial or ethnic group(s) you think the characters involved in the action belong to as soon as you get a mental picture of the group(s).

    a. While I stop at a gas station in the country to fill my car with gas, a pick-up truck stops at a gas tank near mine. I notice an emblem of a Confederate flag on the truck and a gun on the dashboard. A man with a large belly and a tattoo on his right arm gets out of the pick-up and yells, "Hey boy, fill'er up!"

    b. I'm sitting in the family room in a house. The children are polite and well behaved. They bow when the grandfather enters the room and treat him with considerable respect. The children indicate we're having rice for dinner. They are setting the table and ask whether I want a fork or chopsticks.

    c. While walking down an inner-city street, I observe some people sitting in front of a housing project listening to loud music and occasionally getting up to perform some fancy dance steps. A Cadillac stops in front of the project, and an attractive woman gets out. I hear someone say to her, "What's happenin', Momma?"

    d. I'm sitting in the dining room at a table. Several other people are seated around the table, and they're having a great time—drinking wine, eating spaghetti, and laughing loudly. There is opera music playing softly in the background.

2. Probable responses to the vignettes listed above are: (a) poor white; (b) Chinese or other Asian; (c) African American; and (d) Italian. Discuss the following questions:

   a. Were your images and responses based on stereotypes?
   b. How are such stereotypes learned?
   c. When are stereotypes useful? When are they destructive?

3. Read the following "actual" events in each vignette.

   a. The pick-up truck driver is a Native American who borrowed his friend's truck to pick up her daughter, a junior at the university, at the airport. She's studying to be a genetic engineer. The gas station attendant is the man's nephew, an honor student in high school. He is working at the gas station to earn money for college. The man loves his nephew, and the greeting "Hey boy, fill'er up" is his way of relating to his nephew in a loving, joking manner.
   b. The grandfather entering the room is attending his seventy-fifth birthday party. He is a person of German descent who loves Chinese food. He worked as an engineer in Taiwan for a number of years and is adept with chopsticks.
   c. The people sitting on the steps are of Hispanic descent and are preparing for a neighborhood block party. Some of the young people doing "fancy dance steps" are high school students who belong to a folk dance group that will be performing at the block party. The attractive woman stepping out of the Cadillac is the mayor, an Anglo woman who has been invited to the party. The young person who says, "What's happenin', Momma?" does so as a friendly joke. The mayor is sponsoring three children in a South American country by sending them money every month.
   d. The family is an African American family that loves pasta and wine. This is a close-knit, three-generation family. Members enjoy each other and laugh at each other's jokes. The hostess hates loud music while visiting with the relatives, so she turns down the CD player.

4. After you have read the "real" stories, discuss the following questions:

   a. Does the exercise demonstrate that you hold stereotypes?
   b. Do negative stereotypes about ethnic or racial groups lead to prejudice and discrimination?
   c. How can we identify the negative stereotypes we hold so that we do not discriminate against members of the groups that we negatively stereotype?

Competencies/Practice Behaviors Exercise 5.2
Identifying My Prejudices and Stereotypes

Focus Competencies or Practice Behaviors:

- EP 2.1.1b Practice personal reflection and self-correction to assure continual professional development
- EP 2.1.4a Recognize the extent to which a culture's structures and values may oppress, marginalize, alienate, or create or enhance privilege and power

- EP 2.1.4b Gain sufficient self-awareness to eliminate the influence of personal biases and values in working with diverse groups
- EP 2.1.5a Understand forms and mechanisms of oppression and discrimination

A. Brief description

Identify racial and ethnic groups into which you would hesitate to marry, and list reasons for your choices.

B. Objective

You will:

1. Become aware that you hold certain racist and ethnic stereotypes that you need to be aware of in order to develop an objective approach to social work practice with diverse groups.

C. Procedures

1. Since we have been raised in a society in which racist and ethnocentric beliefs flourish, it is likely that we have some racial and ethnic prejudices. It is important that these beliefs be identified. A person who is aware of them can take steps to remain objective in interactions with members of other racial and ethnic groups.
2. The following questionnaire is distributed:

> Assume that you are single. Place an X by the name of each group into which you would hesitate to marry. Do not write your name on this sheet, so that you will remain anonymous.

_____	Russian	_____	White American
_____	Cuban	_____	Arab
_____	French	_____	Israeli
_____	Mexican	_____	Chinese
_____	African American	_____	Japanese
_____	Native American	_____	Filipino
_____	Puerto Rican	_____	Eskimo
_____	Italian	_____	Brazilian
_____	German	_____	Hungarian
_____	Polish	_____	Vietnamese
_____	Norwegian	_____	Pakistani
_____	Samoan	_____	Korean

3. After you complete the first step, write (in the space following the groups that you checked) the reasons why you would hesitate to marry those that you have indicated. This is the part of the exercise that is important in identifying the specific stereotypes you hold. Go beyond writing something like "My parents wouldn't approve" or "I can't see myself marrying such a person" to include the reasons your parents wouldn't approve or the reasons why you can't see yourself marrying such a person.
4. Hand in your responses anonymously. The instructor will read many of the responses to the class. Discuss what a person needs to do to remain objective in interactions with members of ethnic and racial groups about which he or she has negative stereotypes.

Competencies/Practice Behaviors Exercise 5.3
Star Track to New Venus Role-Play

Focus Competencies or Practice Behaviors:

- EP 2.1.1b Practice personal reflection and self-correction to assure continual professional development
- EP 2.1.4a Recognize the extent to which a culture's structures and values may oppress, marginalize, alienate, or create or enhance privilege and power
- EP 2.1.4b Gain sufficient self-awareness to eliminate the influence of personal biases and values in working with diverse groups
- EP 2.1.5a Understand forms and mechanisms of oppression and discrimination

A. Brief description

You will form subgroups. Each subgroup has the task of selecting ethnic and racial groups to continue the human race on a new planet.

B. Objective

You will:

1. Identify some of your positive and negative stereotypes about various racial and ethnic groups.

C. Procedures

1. Form subgroups of about five persons. The instructor reads the following to the subgroups.

> You are living in the year 2013. In 2010, the United States discovered a planet in a distant galaxy that appears to have a climate and atmosphere remarkably similar to Earth's. Scientists are virtually assured this planet, named New Venus, can support human life. In 2011 the United States began building a new spaceship, named *Star Track*, that will be capable of transporting 20 people to New Venus. *Star Track* has recently been completed. In the year 2013 a new comet, Dark Vadim, is discovered, and found to be headed on a collision course for Earth. Scientists predict it will strike at the end of this year. A huge explosion, much worse than a nuclear war, is expected, and many scientists are predicting Earth will disintegrate. The president of the United States has commissioned your subgroup to choose the ethnic and racial backgrounds of the twenty people who will soon board *Star Track* to fly to New Venus in order to continue the human race. The president informs your subgroup that it may select the racial and ethnic backgrounds from the following list. Everyone may come from one ethnic or racial background or from a variety of backgrounds. After you provide your selections, the president will select, consistent with your choices, people in their twenties, including ten men and ten women. All the people selected will be fluent in the English language.
>
> Chinese
> Japanese
> Vietnamese
> Filipino
> Irish
> Egyptian
> German
> French
> Polish
> Hungarian
> Portuguese
> Italian

White American	Saudi Arabian
African American	Iranian
Israeli	Eskimo
Native American	Cuban
Puerto Rican	Australian
Pakistani	Hawaiian
Mexican	Russian

2. While you are making your choices, the instructor lists the names of the racial and ethnic groups on the chalkboard. After you are finished, a representative from each subgroup marks its choices on the board.
3. State the reasons for your choices and why you did not choose people from the racial and ethnic backgrounds that you excluded.
4. The instructor summarizes racial and ethnic stereotypes that are expressed and may end the exercise by asking you what you feel you learned.

Competencies/Practice Behaviors Exercise 5.4
Stranded in Komsa, Russia

Focus Competencies or Practice Behaviors:

- EP 2.1.1b Practice personal reflection and self-correction to assure continual professional development
- EP 2.1.4a Recognize the extent to which a culture's structures and values may oppress, marginalize, alienate, or create or enhance privilege and power
- EP 2.1.4b Gain sufficient self-awareness to eliminate the influence of personal biases and values in working with diverse groups
- EP 2.1.5a Understand forms and mechanisms of oppression and discrimination
- EP 2.1.5b Advocate for human rights and social and economic justice
- EP 2.1.5c Engage in practices that advance social and economic justice

A. Brief description

You will visualize your fears about being stranded in the middle of Russia.

B. Objectives

You will:

1. Understand how racial and ethnic groups feel about living in a country that has oppressed them.

C. Procedures

1. Visualize the following:

You have a passport and are traveling alone by train in Russia. You have a number of exhilarating experiences. The train stops in Komsa, in the heart of Russia, far from any major city. Komsa is a medium-sized city, and you decide to spend a few days in this area. On your first day of shopping and sightseeing, you lose your passport, all your money and traveler's checks, and all your identification. You had all of these in your backpack. You think someone may have stolen these important documents from you, but you don't know who, nor do you know where it happened. You are aware that there is no American embassy in Komsa.

2. The instructor asks the class the following questions. Discuss each question.
   a. If this happened to you, what would be your fears?
   b. To whom would you turn for help?
   c. Do you fear you may be discriminated against or victimized because you are an American?
   d. Are the fears and concerns that you have similar to the concerns of racial and ethnic minorities who live in a country where the majority group has a history of discriminating against them?
   e. If you were a worker at a social welfare agency that is identified with the white power structure in our society, how might you seek to reduce the fears and concerns that nonwhite clients may have in asking for help?

Competencies/Practice Behaviors Exercise 5.5
Multicultural Sensitivity

Focus Competencies or Practice Behaviors:

- EP 2.1.1b Practice personal reflection and self-correction to assure continual professional development
- EP 2.1.4a Recognize the extent to which a culture's structures and values may oppress, marginalize, alienate, or create or enhance privilege and power
- EP 2.1.4b Gain sufficient self-awareness to eliminate the influence of personal biases and values in working with diverse groups
- EP 2.1.5a Understand forms and mechanisms of oppression and discrimination

A. Brief description

A cultural sensitivity test is administered. It is designed to test your knowledge of several diverse cultural groups. Understanding diverse cultures is essential for effective work with clients.

B. Objectives

You will:

1. Examine your own levels of understanding of some basic aspects of several diverse cultures.
2. Recognize the importance of learning more about cultures that may be different from your own.

C. Procedure

1. The following questions are designed to test your understanding of some important aspects of four diverse cultural groups. Answer them to the best of your ability.

A. AFRICAN AMERICAN CULTURAL DIFFERENCES TEST

1. What does NAACP stand for?

2. In what year was NAACP established?
   a. 1865
   b. 1889
   c. 1909
   d. 1935

3. What does NABSW stand for and when was it established?

4. How does African American music express African American culture?

5. When did slavery end?

6. Kwanzaa is:
   a. A starchy grain originally imported by African slaves abducted in West Africa.
   b. An African American festival held in late December.
   c. An African American dance.
   d. A Muslim prayer sequence originally brought from Africa by abducted slaves.

Note: Donnise Bartholomew, Holly Lambert, Stephan Jurgen, Johnathan Greene, Geri McKinney, Nicole Leonard, Tameka Hinton, Janet Bonvillian, Lili Largent, and Rufus Brown, all social work majors at Clark Atlanta University, suggested questions #1, #5, and #6 on this test.

B. CHICANO CULTURAL DIFFERENCES

1. The Treaty of Guadalupe Hildago ceded to the United States what is now known as:
   a. The state of Texas
   b. The state of New Mexico
   c. The state of California
   d. The southwestern United States

2. Cinco de Mayo is a Mexican holiday that commemorates:
   a. Mexico's independence from France
   b. The battle of Puebla
   c. The death of the Frito Bandito
   d. The decline of the Diaz regime

3. A "frajo" is a:
   a. Short handled hoe
   b. Car
   c. Cigarette
   d. Pachuco

4. A "curandera" is a:
   a. Healer
   b. Witch
   c. Curious person

5. The 12th of December is:
   a. Cesar Chavez's birthday
   b. The day of the Virgin of Guadalupe
   c. The anniversary of "pachuco" riots

6. To Chicanos, the term "carnal" means:
   a. Brother
   b. Butcher
   c. Sports car
   d. Enemy

7. A "tio taco" is:
   a. A Mexican dish
   b. An individual who rejects his culture
   c. A Cuban
   d. An uncle from Spain

8. The most valued institution in Chicano culture is:
   a. The school
   b. The church
   c. The government
   d. The family

C. NATIVE AMERICAN CULTURAL DIFFERENCES

1. Which of the following is <u>not</u> a Native American invention?
   a. Canoe
   b. Kayak
   c. Parka
   d. Tomahawk

2. The words "Kemo sabe," popularized by the Lone Ranger's sidekick, Tonto, mean:
   a. White Friend
   b. Blue Eyes
   c. Honky
   d. Nothing at all

3. The phrase "The only good Indian is a dead Indian" is attributed to:
   a. Gen. Philip Sheridan
   b. Gen. Wm. T. Sherman
   c. Col. Henry B. Carrington
   d. Lt. Col. George A. Custer

4. Which of the following was not a member of the League of Six Nations (Iroquois Confederacy)?
   a. Oneida
   b. Seneca
   c. Kiowa
   d. Onondaga

5. Which of the following colleges was first instituted primarily to educate Indians?
   a. Yale
   b. Harvard
   c. Dartmouth
   d. Princeton

D. ASIAN CULTURAL DIFFERENCES

1. Buddha-Dharma is ____
   a. The teachings of Judo
   b. The practice of Oriental cooking
   c. The teachings of the Buddha
   d. The wife of the Buddha

2. The art of bonsai refers to ____
   a. Japanese silk screening
   b. Chinese wrestling
   c. Growing miniature trees
   d. None of the above

3. The "koto" is ____
   a. A Korean word for house
   b. A thirteen-string Japanese musical instrument
   c. The newest Oriental dance to hit the West Coast
   d. The Vietnamese national anthem

4. Which word sometimes means a Japanese ghetto? ____
   a. Nihon machi
   b. Sakana
   c. Kanji
   d. Ghettuloheli

5. Third generation Japanese are called ____
   a. Issei
   b. Nisei
   c. Yonsei
   d. Sansei

A. ANSWERS TO THE AFRICAN AMERICAN CULTURAL DIFFERENCES TEST:

1. National Association for the Advancement of Colored People
2. c
3. National Association of Black Social Workers, 1968
4. African American music expresses African American culture as it "represents the combining of African characteristics with the content and conditions of being Black in the United States;" additionally, it "is a concrete demonstration of culture as dynamic and changing with African musical characteristics and Afro-American musical forms incorporating new technology (i.e., brass and piano) after the Civil War and creating additional Afro-American musical forms (i.e., blues, jazz, gospel)". (This question was posed and answered by Jualynne E. Dodson in *An Afrocentric Educational Manual: Toward a Non-Deficit Perspective in Services to Families and Children* [Knoxville: University of Tennessee School of Social Work Office of Continuing Social Work Education, 1983], 57)
5. "The Civil War began in 1861, and on January 1, 1863, President Abraham Lincoln issued the Emancipation Proclamation, proclaiming that all slaves would be free. With the defeat of the Confederate army, slavery was ultimately made illegal in 1865 with the adoption of the 13th amendment" (Bogart R. Leashore, "African Americans Overview" in *The Encyclopedia of Social Work*, 19th ed. (Washington, D.C.: National Association of Social Workers Press, 1995), 103)
6. b (*Webster's Ninth New Collegiate Dictionary* (Springfield, MA: Mirriam-Webster, 1991), 667)

B. ANSWERS TO CHICANO CULTURAL DIFFERENCES TEST:

1. (d) The treaty of Guadalupe Hildago was signed by the United States and Mexico in 1848. With this treaty, Mexico accepted the Rio Grande as the Texas border and ceded the Southwest (which incorporates the present-day states of Arizona, California, New Mexico, Utah, Nevada, and parts of Colorado) to the United States in return for $15 million.

2. (b) This celebration commemorates a battle in which a small Mexican army defeated a French army battalion. Cinco de Mayo celebrations are still held in Mexico and in the United States where there are a significant number of Chicanos.

3. (c) The term "frajo" is a slang word for cigarette, which is commonly used in the barrio.

4. (a) The "curandera" is a person who is able to relieve people of their physical sickness. Many elderly Chicano people do not believe in the "doctor" as they are known in this country. They prefer to be attended by the curandera, or healer.

5. (b) Chicanos are a very religious people. The 12th of December is the day of the patron saint of the Chicano people—the Virgin of Guadalupe.

6. (a) "Carnal" means brother. It is usually used as a greeting between males.

7. (b) Many individuals reject their culture due to the educational system in this country. Chicanos have been taught that their culture is inferior and that the Anglo-American culture is superior. Therefore, many Mexican Americans (especially second and third generation) do not identify with their cultural heritage and the term "Chicano."

8. (d) Chicano families are traditionally very, very close. The total Chicano existence revolves around the family.

C. ANSWERS TO THE NATIVE AMERICAN DIFFERENCES TEST:

1. (d) The tomahawk was a French invention later copied and used extensively by Native Americans.

2. (d) No one knows where this phrase comes from; there are no known languages that this can be traced to—it's another Hollywood gimmick.

3. (a) Gen. Sheridan's direct quote: "The only good Indians I ever saw were dead." The phrase was later simplified.

4. (c) The Six Nations was composed of: Oneida, Seneca, Tuscarora, Onondaga, Cayuga, and Mohawk.

5. (c) Dartmouth.

D. ANSWERS TO THE ASIAN CULTURAL DIFFERENCES TEST:

1. c
2. c
3. b
4. a
5. d

2. Discuss reactions to the test. You can begin with the following questions:
   a. How easy or difficult was it to answer these questions?
   b. How did you feel when you didn't know the answers?
   c. Were any of the answers surprising to you and, if so, which ones? Explain why.
   d. How might your ignorance of these and other significant aspects of a diverse culture hinder your work with clients in that cultural group?
   e. What concrete steps can you take to enhance your knowledge of various cultural groups?

Chapter 5 Competencies/Practice Behaviors Exercises Assessment:

Name: ______________________________ **Date:** __________
Supervisor's Name: ______________________________

Focus Competencies or Practice Behaviors:

- EP 2.1.1b Practice personal reflection and self-correction to assure continual professional development
- EP 2.1.4a Recognize the extent to which a culture's structures and values may oppress, marginalize, alienate, or create or enhance privilege and power
- EP 2.1.4b Gain sufficient self-awareness to eliminate the influence of personal biases and values in working with diverse groups
- EP 2.1.5a Understand forms and mechanisms of oppression and discrimination
- EP 2.1.5b Advocate for human rights and social and economic justice
- EP 2.1.5c Engage in practices that advance social and economic justice

Instructions:

A. Evaluate your work or your partner's work in the Focus Competencies/Practice Behaviors by completing the Competencies/Practice Behaviors Assessment form below

B. What other Competencies/Practice Behaviors did you use to complete these Exercises? Be sure to record them in your assessments

1.	I have attained this competency/practice behavior (in the range of 81 to 100%)
2.	I have largely attained this competency/practice behavior (in the range of 61 to 80%)
3.	I have partially attained this competency/practice behavior (in the range of 41 to 60%)
4.	I have made a little progress in attaining this competency/practice behavior (in the range of 21 to 40%)
5.	I have made almost no progress in attaining this competency/practice behavior (in the range of 0 to 20%)

EPAS 2008 Core Competencies & Core Practice Behaviors	Student Self Assessment						Evaluator Feedback
Student and Evaluator Assessment Scale and Comments	**0**	**1**	**2**	**3**	**4**	**5**	**Agree/Disagree/Comments**
EP 2.1.1 Identify as a Professional Social Worker and Conduct Oneself Accordingly:							
a. Advocate for client access to the services of social work							
b. Practice personal reflection and self-correction to assure continual professional development							
c. Attend to professional roles and boundaries							
d. Demonstrate professional demeanor in behavior, appearance, and communication							
e. Engage in career-long learning							
f. Use supervision and consultation							
EP 2.1.2 Apply Social Work Ethical Principles to Guide Professional Practice:							
a. Recognize and manage personal values in a way that allows professional values to guide practice							

b. Make ethical decisions by applying NASW Code of Ethics and, as applicable, of the IFSW/IASSW Ethics in Social Work, Statement of Principles							
c. Tolerate ambiguity in resolving ethical conflicts							
d. Apply strategies of ethical reasoning to arrive at principled decisions							
EP 2.1.3 Apply Critical Thinking to Inform and Communicate Professional Judgments:							
a. Distinguish, appraise, and integrate multiple sources of knowledge, including research-based knowledge and practice wisdom							
b. Analyze models of assessment, prevention, intervention, and evaluation							
c. Demonstrate effective oral and written communication in working with individuals, families, groups, organizations, communities, and colleagues							
EP 2.1.4 Engage Diversity and Difference in Practice:							
a. Recognize the extent to which a culture's structures and values may oppress, marginalize, alienate, or create or enhance privilege and power							
b. Gain sufficient self-awareness to eliminate the influence of personal biases and values in working with diverse groups							
c. Recognize and communicate their understanding of the importance of difference in shaping life experiences							
d. View themselves as learners and engage those with whom they work as informants							
EP 2.1.5 Advance Human Rights and Social and Economic Justice:							
a. Understand forms and mechanisms of oppression and discrimination							
b. Advocate for human rights and social and economic justice							
c. Engage in practices that advance social and economic justice							
EP 2.1.6 Engage in Research-Informed Practice and Practice-Informed Research:							
a. Use practice experience to inform scientific inquiry							
b. Use research evidence to inform practice							
EP 2.1.7 Apply Knowledge of Human Behavior and the Social Environment:							
a. Utilize conceptual frameworks to guide the processes of assessment, intervention, and evaluation							
b. Critique and apply knowledge to understand person and environment							
EP 2.1.8 Engage in Policy Practice to Advance Social and Economic Well-Being and to Deliver Effective Social Work Services:							
a. Analyze, formulate, and advocate for policies that advance social well-being							
b. Collaborate with colleagues and clients for effective policy action							

EP 2.1.9 Respond to Contexts that Shape Practice:							
a. Continuously discover, appraise, and attend to changing locales, populations, scientific and technological developments, and emerging societal trends to provide relevant services							
b. Provide leadership in promoting sustainable changes in service delivery and practice to improve the quality of social services							
EP 2.1.10 Engage, Assess, Intervene, and Evaluate with Individuals, Families, Groups, Organizations and Communities:							
a. Substantively and affectively prepare for action with individuals, families, groups, organizations, and communities							
b. Use empathy and other interpersonal skills							
c. Develop a mutually agreed-on focus of work and desired outcomes							
d. Collect, organize, and interpret client data							
e. Assess client strengths and limitations							
f. Develop mutually agreed-on intervention goals and objectives							
g. Select appropriate intervention strategies							
h. Initiate actions to achieve organizational goals							
i. Implement prevention interventions that enhance client capacities							
j. Help clients resolve problems							
k. Negotiate, mediate, and advocate for clients							
l. Facilitate transitions and endings							
m. Critically analyze, monitor, and evaluate interventions							

Chapter 6
Biological Development in Adolescence

Competencies/Practice Behaviors Exercise 6.1
Self-Portrait

Focus Competencies or Practice Behaviors:

- EP 2.1.1b Practice personal reflection and self-correction to assure continual professional development
- EP 2.1.7b Critique and apply knowledge to understand person and environment
- EP 2.1.10a Substantively and affectively prepare for action with individuals, families, groups, organizations, and communities
- EP 2.1.10b Use empathy and other interpersonal skills

A. Brief description

Draw a picture of yourself as an adolescent and examine your own perceived physical strengths and weaknesses. Small-group discussions and a large-group discussion follow.

B. Objectives

You will:

1. Identify specific areas of concern that you had when you were an adolescent.
2. Relate these concerns to the concerns of adolescents in general.
3. Examine the impacts of physical changes and the perceptions of these changes on the individual personality.
4. Relate the physical changes you experienced to the factual material presented in the text.

C. Procedure

1. You are given a sheet of paper and asked to draw a clothed illustration of yourself at age 13 in the center.
2. Label the upper-left-hand portion of the paper "Strengths" and the upper-right-hand portion "Weaknesses." List under the appropriate headings both the positive physical aspects and the negative physical aspects you perceived yourself to have at age 13.
3. Divide into groups of four to six persons. Discuss at least some of the physical strengths and weaknesses you perceived in yourself during adolescence. You will have approximately 10 minutes for this discussion.
4. Small groups come together for a large-group discussion. The large group considers the following questions:
   a. What does it feel like to be an adolescent?
   b. What specific physical changes tend to be the most striking and have the greatest effects on the developing personality?
   c. How do these physical changes and their effects on individual personalities relate to the research and factual material presented in the text? On what issues did the small groups and the text agree? Where were there differences?

Competencies/Practice Behaviors Exercise 6.2
The Birth Control Dilemma Role-Play

Focus Competencies or Practice Behaviors:

- EP 2.1.1b Practice personal reflection and self-correction to assure continual professional development
- EP 2.1.2a Recognize and manage personal values in a way that allows professional values to guide practice
- EP 2.1.9a Continuously discover, appraise, and attend to changing locales, populations, scientific and technological developments, and emerging societal trends to provide relevant services
- EP 2.1.10a Substantively and affectively prepare for action with individuals, families, groups, organizations, and communities
- EP 2.1.10b Use empathy and other interpersonal skills
- EP 2.1.10g Select appropriate intervention strategies

A. Brief description

You will choose a partner; one person plays a social worker and the other a 16-year-old adolescent trying to decide what type of contraception to use. Various alternatives, and their strengths and weaknesses, are examined during the role-play. A group discussion follows.

B. Objectives

You will:

1. Identify the various methods of contraception.
2. Assess the positive and negative aspects of each.
3. Examine steps in decision making about means of contraception to use.
4. Recognize the differences between personal opinion and professional objectivity.
5. Examine your own values and opinions concerning birth control.

C. Procedure

1. Review the various methods of birth control presented in the text and the advantages and disadvantages of each.
2. Write down your personal opinion about which method of contraception is best. There is <u>no one best method</u>; the choice is personal.
3. Choose a partner; one person role-plays a 16-year-old adolescent and the other an adult acquaintance of that adolescent.

> **IF THE ADOLESCENT IS A FEMALE:** Frankie is 15 years old and confused. She has been going steady with Johnnie for four months now. Two weeks ago they started having sexual intercourse. They have not been using any form of birth control. Although Frankie has avoided admitting it to herself, she has finally accepted the fact that she is sexually active. She's afraid of getting pregnant and wants to use some form of birth control. The problem is that she doesn't know which one to use. She goes to an adult she knows and whom she trusts will keep their conversation confidential. She asks the adult what the best form of birth control would be for her to use.

IF THE ADOLESCENT IS A MALE: Focus attention on Johnnie, the 16-year-old boyfriend. Everything about the role-play remains the same except for the fact that it is the male in the couple who is seeking birth-control advice.

4. Review the basic suggestions for doing a role-play. The adult role-player is not a professional social worker or counselor but only a friend who can give information and ask questions. The adult role-players:
   a. Ask the adolescent what he or she knows about birth-control methods.
   b. Provide information about forms of contraception available.
   c. Help the adolescent examine the pros and cons of each birth-control alternative and come to a final decision about what type to use.
   d. Remember that choosing a birth-control method is the adolescent's decision. Try to be objective.
5. You will have 10 to 15 minutes to complete the role-plays. Pairs role-play simultaneously.
6. Class discussion follows the role-playing:
   a. How did the adolescent and the adult differ in their views of "the best" method of birth control?
   b. What advantages and disadvantages of the various methods were most important to the adolescent?
   c. How did the adult role-players feel when their views differed from the adolescent's feelings about various contraceptive methods?
   d. How did the adolescent arrive at a final decision concerning what type of contraception to use?

Competencies/Practice Behaviors Exercise 6.3
How Did You First Learn About Sex?

Focus Competencies or Practice Behaviors:

- EP 2.1.1b Practice personal reflection and self-correction to assure continual professional development
- EP 2.1.3a Distinguish, appraise, and integrate multiple sources of knowledge, including research-based knowledge and practice wisdom
- EP 2.1.7b Critique and apply knowledge to understand person and environment
- EP 2.1.8a Analyze, formulate, and advocate for policies that advance social well-being

A. Brief description

The group is broken down into smaller groups of four to six. The small groups are asked to discuss how individual members first learned about sex. Major points of each group's discussion and the total group's discussion are summarized.

B. Objectives

You will:

1. Identify and describe the circumstances under which you first learned about sex.
2. Explore the issue of how comfortable parents feel providing sex education to their children.
3. Examine the need for sex education and relate it to your own experience.

C. Procedure
1. Form groups of four to six members. Select a group of people with whom you feel at ease.
2. Address the following questions:
    a. How did you first learn about sex? What were the circumstances? Who was it that talked to you about it?
    b. How comfortable did your parents feel discussing sex with you?
    c. What kind of sex education did you receive in school?
    d. What is your opinion about the need for sex education?
3. You have 10 to 15 minutes to discuss the questions.
4. One representative of each group summarizes that group's discussion and shares this summary with the larger group.
5. Finally, formulate a summary statement regarding the conclusions of the entire class.

Competencies/Practice Behaviors Exercise 6.4
Sex Education for an Adolescent Role-Play

Focus Competencies or Practice Behaviors:
- EP 2.1.1b Practice personal reflection and self-correction to assure continual professional development
- EP 2.1.3c Demonstrate effective oral and written communication in working with individuals, families, groups, organizations, communities, and colleagues
- EP 2.1.7b Critique and apply knowledge to understand person and environment

A. Brief description
The instructor will role-play an adolescent and ask the entire class to respond to questions.

B. Objectives
You will:
1. Identify gaps in basic sexual information given to adolescents.
2. Appraise your own levels of sexual knowledge and formulate answers to questions in a simulated situation.
3. Recognize the difficulty of sharing sexual information clearly and simply.
4. Examine your own ability to talk about sexual issues.

C. Procedure
1. The instructor role-plays a 14-year-old adolescent who asks various questions about sex.
2. Class members call out the answers.
3. Questions asked may include the following:
    a. When is the right time to start having sex?
    b. Can boys pull out in time?
    c. What does an orgasm feel like?
    d. Does it hurt the first time you have sex?
    e. Can a person get any STIs from oral sex? If so, what kinds?
    f. What do boys want?
    g. What do girls want?
4. The instructor responds to group members' answers as an adolescent might. Group members' words should be clear and simple. Explanations should be specific.
5. Discuss your reactions to the experience.

Chapter 6 Competencies/Practice Behaviors Exercises Assessment:

Name: ______________________ **Date:** __________
Supervisor's Name: ______________________

Focus Competencies or Practice Behaviors:

- EP 2.1.1b Practice personal reflection and self-correction to assure continual professional development
- EP 2.1.2a Recognize and manage personal values in a way that allows professional values to guide practice
- EP 2.1.3a Distinguish, appraise, and integrate multiple sources of knowledge, including research-based knowledge and practice wisdom
- EP 2.1.3c Demonstrate effective oral and written communication in working with individuals, families, groups, organizations, communities, and colleagues
- EP 2.1.7b Critique and apply knowledge to understand person and environment
- EP 2.1.8a Analyze, formulate, and advocate for policies that advance social well-being
- EP 2.1.9a Continuously discover, appraise, and attend to changing locales, populations, scientific and technological developments, and emerging societal trends to provide relevant services
- EP 2.1.10a Substantively and affectively prepare for action with individuals, families, groups, organizations, and communities
- EP 2.1.10b Use empathy and other interpersonal skills
- EP 2.1.10g Select appropriate intervention strategies

Instructions:

A. Evaluate your work or your partner's work in the Focus Competencies/Practice Behaviors by completing the Competencies/Practice Behaviors Assessment form below

B. What other Competencies/Practice Behaviors did you use to complete these Exercises? Be sure to record them in your assessments

1.	I have attained this competency/practice behavior (in the range of 81 to 100%)
2.	I have largely attained this competency/practice behavior (in the range of 61 to 80%)
3.	I have partially attained this competency/practice behavior (in the range of 41 to 60%)
4.	I have made a little progress in attaining this competency/practice behavior (in the range of 21 to 40%)
5.	I have made almost no progress in attaining this competency/practice behavior (in the range of 0 to 20%)

EPAS 2008 Core Competencies & Core Practice Behaviors	Student Self Assessment						Evaluator Feedback
Student and Evaluator Assessment Scale and Comments	0	1	2	3	4	5	Agree/Disagree/Comments
EP 2.1.1 Identify as a Professional Social Worker and Conduct Oneself Accordingly:							
a. Advocate for client access to the services of social work							
b. Practice personal reflection and self-correction to assure continual professional development							
c. Attend to professional roles and boundaries							

d. Demonstrate professional demeanor in behavior, appearance, and communication							
e. Engage in career-long learning							
f. Use supervision and consultation							
EP 2.1.2 Apply Social Work Ethical Principles to Guide Professional Practice:							
a. Recognize and manage personal values in a way that allows professional values to guide practice							
b. Make ethical decisions by applying NASW Code of Ethics and, as applicable, of the IFSW/IASSW Ethics in Social Work, Statement of Principles							
c. Tolerate ambiguity in resolving ethical conflicts							
d. Apply strategies of ethical reasoning to arrive at principled decisions							
EP 2.1.3 Apply Critical Thinking to Inform and Communicate Professional Judgments:							
a. Distinguish, appraise, and integrate multiple sources of knowledge, including research-based knowledge and practice wisdom							
b. Analyze models of assessment, prevention, intervention, and evaluation							
c. Demonstrate effective oral and written communication in working with individuals, families, groups, organizations, communities, and colleagues							
EP 2.1.4 Engage Diversity and Difference in Practice:							
a. Recognize the extent to which a culture's structures and values may oppress, marginalize, alienate, or create or enhance privilege and power							
b. Gain sufficient self-awareness to eliminate the influence of personal biases and values in working with diverse groups							
c. Recognize and communicate their understanding of the importance of difference in shaping life experiences							
d. View themselves as learners and engage those with whom they work as informants							
EP 2.1.5 Advance Human Rights and Social and Economic Justice:							
a. Understand forms and mechanisms of oppression and discrimination							
b. Advocate for human rights and social and economic justice							
c. Engage in practices that advance social and economic justice							
EP 2.1.6 Engage in Research-Informed Practice and Practice-Informed Research:							
a. Use practice experience to inform scientific inquiry							
b. Use research evidence to inform practice							
EP 2.1.7 Apply Knowledge of Human Behavior and the Social Environment:							
a. Utilize conceptual frameworks to guide the processes of assessment, intervention, and evaluation							

b. Critique and apply knowledge to understand person and environment							
EP 2.1.8 Engage in Policy Practice to Advance Social and Economic Well-Being and to Deliver Effective Social Work Services:							
a. Analyze, formulate, and advocate for policies that advance social well-being							
b. Collaborate with colleagues and clients for effective policy action							
EP 2.1.9 Respond to Contexts that Shape Practice:							
a. Continuously discover, appraise, and attend to changing locales, populations, scientific and technological developments, and emerging societal trends to provide relevant services							
b. Provide leadership in promoting sustainable changes in service delivery and practice to improve the quality of social services							
EP 2.1.10 Engage, Assess, Intervene, and Evaluate with Individuals, Families, Groups, Organizations and Communities:							
a. Substantively and affectively prepare for action with individuals, families, groups, organizations, and communities							
b. Use empathy and other interpersonal skills							
c. Develop a mutually agreed-on focus of work and desired outcomes							
d. Collect, organize, and interpret client data							
e. Assess client strengths and limitations							
f. Develop mutually agreed-on intervention goals and objectives							
g. Select appropriate intervention strategies							
h. Initiate actions to achieve organizational goals							
i. Implement prevention interventions that enhance client capacities							
j. Help clients resolve problems							
k. Negotiate, mediate, and advocate for clients							
l. Facilitate transitions and endings							
m. Critically analyze, monitor, and evaluate interventions							

Chapter 7
Psychological Development in Adolescence

Competencies/Practice Behaviors Exercise 7.1
Assessment of Suicide Potential

Focus Competencies or Practice Behaviors:

- EP 2.1.4c Recognize and communicate their understanding of the importance of difference in shaping life experiences
- EP 2.1.7a Utilize conceptual frameworks to guide the processes of assessment, intervention, and evaluation
- EP 2.1.7b Critique and apply knowledge to understand person and environment
- EP 2.1.10a Substantively and affectively prepare for action with individuals, families, groups, organizations, and communities

A. Brief description

Two vignettes describing depressed people are presented. You will evaluate the suicide potential of each person on the basis of the SAD PERSONS scale.

B. Objectives

You will:

1. Recognize the variables that contribute to suicide potential.
2. Apply knowledge about suicide potential to lifelike situations.

C. Procedure

1. Review the material concerning suicide presented in the text. Examine carefully each variable described by the SAD PERSONS scale.
2. The instructor presents the following descriptions of potentially suicidal persons. These may be role-played or simply read by the instructor. After each vignette, you may ask further questions about the potentially suicidal person. These questions may be answered arbitrarily with any information the instructor wishes to include.

a. Jerome, age 18, is depressed. He lives in one of the poor, inner city, African American neighborhoods of a large urban area. He finished high school, in a way. Reading and writing are not really some of his strengths. He managed to slip through each grade because he had a knack for playing basketball. He wasn't quite good enough for playing in the pros or even in college, but he had been good enough to play on the high school varsity team. Sports and connections with his family helped to keep him out of gang involvement.

Jerome is also bored. He has looked everywhere for a job but just can't find anything. He almost landed one as a janitor at a local supermarket. However, one of the prior employees returned to the city and got it instead. Even that job only paid minimum wage. It was hardly enough to move out of his parents' home and live on his own.

That's another thing. All his parents seem to do lately is nag. They want him to get out and do something useful. He tries to tell them how hard he has been looking for a job, but they don't seem to understand. His father has been working at a local clothing store for years. Jerome's family is poor but certainly not starving. His parents are also disappointed that he didn't go on to college. They have been hoping that Jerome's life would be better than their own in terms of opportunity and financial security.

Now Jerome has given up. The only thing left to do, it seems, is to sit around some of the local bars and drink with his old buddies who are in similar situations. How depressing. Lately, Jerome is considering ending it all. What is the use, anyway? He has no future. Things don't matter. Maybe he will just borrow a friend's old wreck of a car and drive off the Center Street Bridge. One of these days maybe he will do just that—end it all.

b. Susie, age 17, has just started college this semester. She is depressed. All she seems to do is homework. She has opted to attend the major public university in her state. Her choice was based mostly on pressure from her high school steady boyfriend of two years who also wanted to attend this school. It is so big, scary, and lonely. It is also impersonal. She is just a freshman in classes of up to 300 other students. Sometimes she feels as if her entire identity is an identification number. The stark contrast with her high school experience makes it even worse. In high school, she had been very active in extracurricular activities and had scores of friends.

Her grades aren't very good either. She was accustomed to receiving almost straight A's in high school. Here she is barely maintaining a B average. She is taking an accelerated biology course that is baffling her with complicated theories. She is also taking an upper-level Spanish course that seems impossible to master. She might as well be taking ancient Russian. No matter how many hours she works, she can barely maintain a B- average in that course.

Another problem is her boyfriend. She used to think that she really loved him, but he just can't seem to find much time for her these days. He loves school. He is enjoying his studies and making new friends. Lately, whenever they get together, all they seem to do is fight. She is feeling like quite a "bitch" because of her incessant pleading that he give her more of his time.

Loneliness is another problem area. There are two or three people on her dormitory floor with whom she can talk a little and occasionally goes out for pizza. Susie doesn't do much else, though. All the other students seem to be having fun. But then, even if she did have friends, she couldn't do anything with them. She drives herself to study almost every waking hour.

Susie is very close to her family, who live in another city. Several weeks ago, her uncle died suddenly and unexpectedly. She had been very close to him and misses him very much. She knows she shouldn't keep calling her parents and crying to them on the phone about how depressed she is. They have their own problems.

Lately, she has been thinking about killing herself. She has thought about jumping off the top of her 15-story dorm, but she doesn't really know how to get up there. Maybe she can find some poison. Sometimes she thinks about what substances are poisonous. Cleaning fluid and ammonia don't appeal to her very much.

Life is certainly bleak. For Susie it is just too hard to live.

3. Evaluate the person's suicide potential according to the SAD PERSONS scale. Do it silently and write down your conclusions.
4. Discuss the following questions:
   a. How did you rate each person's suicide potential?
   b. What are the similarities and differences in their life situations?
   c. How might you go about trying to help them?

Competencies/Practice Behaviors Exercise 7.2
Forming an Identity

Focus Competencies or Practice Behaviors:

- EP 2.1.1b Practice personal reflection and self-correction to assure continual professional development
- EP 2.1.4b Gain sufficient self-awareness to eliminate the influence of personal biases and values in working with diverse groups
- EP 2.1.4c Recognize and communicate their understanding of the importance of difference in shaping life experiences

A. Brief description

You will answer 18 questions designed to help you arrive at a sense of who you are and what you want out of life.

B. Objectives

You will:

1. Understand that forming a sense of who you are is one of the most important psychological tasks you face.
2. Examine the extent to which you have formulated a personal identity.
3. Identify specific areas you have to focus on in order to formulate a more thorough sense of who you are.

C. Procedure

1. Summarize the text material on the importance of arriving at an identity.
2. Write answers to the questions that appear at the end of this exercise.
3. After you have completed writing answers, the instructor will ask for volunteers to share what they wrote.
4. What questions caused the most struggle? (Some future class periods may be devoted to providing information about these areas.) What do you feel you learned from this process?

FORMING AN IDENTITY: ARRIVING AT A SENSE OF WHO I AM AND WHAT I WANT OUT OF LIFE

1. What do I find satisfying, meaningful, and enjoyable? (Only after you identify what is meaningful and gratifying will you be able to consciously seek involvement in activities that will make your life fulfilling and avoid those activities that are meaningless or stifling.)

2. What is my moral code? (One possible code is to seek to fulfill your needs and to do what you find enjoyable in a way that does not deprive others of the ability to fulfill their needs.)

3. What are my spiritual beliefs?

4. What are my employment goals? (Ideally, you should seek employment that you find stimulating and satisfying, that you are skilled at, and that provides you with enough money to support your lifestyle.)

5. What are my sexual mores? (All of us should develop a consistent code that we are comfortable with and that helps us to meet our needs without exploiting others. There is no one right code—what works for one may not work for another, due to differences in lifestyles, life goals, and personal values.)

6. Do I want to have a committed relationship? (If yes, with what type of person and when? How consistent are your answers here with your other life goals?)

7. Do I desire to have children? (If yes, how many and when? If you already have children, do you want to have more children? How consistent are your answers here with your other life goals?)

8. In what area of the country or world do I want to live? (Variables to be considered are climate, geography, type of dwelling, rural or urban setting, closeness to relatives or friends, and characteristics of the neighborhood.)

9. What do I enjoy doing with my leisure time?

10. What kind of image do I want to project to others? (Your image will be composed of your dressing style and grooming habits, emotions, personality, assertiveness, capacity to communicate, material possessions, moral code, physical features, and voice patterns. You need to assess your strengths and shortcomings honestly in this area and seek to make needed improvements.)

11. What type of people do I enjoy being with, and why?

12. Do I desire to improve the quality of my life and that of others? (If yes, in what ways? How do you hope to achieve these goals?)

13. What types of relationships do I desire to have with relatives, friends, neighbors, and people I meet for the first time?

14. What are my thoughts about death and dying?

15. What are the most severe stresses in my life at the moment?

16. How am I handling these stresses? What strategies am I using to resolve them?

17. What do I want to accomplish in the next 5 years?

18. What are my plans for accomplishing the goals I listed in question 17?

Competencies/Practice Behaviors Exercise 7.3
Are You Assertive Role-Play

Focus Competencies or Practice Behaviors:

- EP 2.1.1b Practice personal reflection and self-correction to assure continual professional development
- EP 2.1.3c Demonstrate effective oral and written communication in working with individuals, families, groups, organizations, communities, and colleagues

A. Brief description

Volunteers will be asked to role-play a series of situations before the entire class. Potentially assertive, nonassertive, and aggressive responses to these situations will be examined and discussed.

B. Objectives

This exercise will enable you to:

1. Recognize assertive, nonassertive, and aggressive responses (both verbal and nonverbal) to problematic situations.
2. Examine the effectiveness of these types of responses.
3. Propose specific effective assertive techniques.

C. Procedure

1. Following are a series of situations, each of which sets the stage for a role-play. In each role-play, two persons are described. One person is either making a request or doing something annoying. Your instructor will ask for two volunteers for each role-play to act out the characters. One volunteer plays the "annoyer." The other volunteer plays a person who's trying to act as assertively as possible in response:

a. Ethel and Fred, both college students, have been dating steadily for the past eighteen months. Typically, they go to a movie or a sporting event on a Friday night and then out for pizza or subs afterward. Ethel really likes Fred and enjoys their evenings out together except for one thing. Every single Friday night while they're eating, Fred says something like, "You know, Ethel, you really shouldn't be eating such fattening food. It looks like you're gaining weight."

The scene is the local pizzeria. Ethel and Fred are midway through their pepperoni, mushroom, and black olive pizza when Fred makes his usual comment.

b. Valerie and Nikki, best friends, are taking an upper-level sociology course that requires voluminous amounts of reading. Most of the reading is from supplementary sources that have been placed on reserve in the college library. Valerie has spent dozens of hours reading the material and taking copious notes in preparation for the upcoming cumulative exam. Nikki, on the other hand, has done some of the work. However, she really feels she isn't much good at taking notes, so she didn't. Nikki's had a good semester and has done a lot of partying. Valerie remembers some of her miserable weekend nights alone in the library while Nikki was out having fun.

The scene is the eve of the exam. Valerie and Nikki go to the library together to study. Nikki bluntly asks Valerie if she can study from the notes Valerie's been taking all semester while reading the reserve materials.

c. Harry is standing in line at Randall's Country Market with a cart full of groceries. It's late Friday afternoon and the market is crowded. There are five people ahead of him in line. He thinks to himself that he has a knack for picking the slowest line possiblc. Harry is in a horrendous hurry as he has dinner reservations in an hour. The reservations were difficult to get and he is looking forward to the event very much. He's thinking how difficult it will be to make it to the restaurant on time. A woman with a crying child in her arms breaks in at the head of the line with a full cart of groceries and says, "Excuse me, but I have to get through."

d. Tim works as a house parent at a group home for adults with developmental disabilities. He's going to school full-time with a social work major, while working at the group home part-time. He's supposed to work three evenings each week from 4:00 p.m. to midnight. He really likes his job and feels it will be good experience and look good on his resume when he gets his degree and looks for a full-time professional position. Sharon, his supervisor, has asked him to work an extra two to three nights each week for the past month. Another worker quit and she hasn't had time to fill the position yet. Tim wants to stay "on her good side" because he knows he will have to depend on her for a good reference someday. Therefore, each time she's asked him to work, he has. The problem is that he's starting to get tired and feels his schoolwork is suffering because of all the extra hours he's been working. Sharon approaches Tim and asks him if he could work an extra two nights next week. She initiates the request by saying how well he does his job and how she can always depend on him.

2. Each role-play should continue for no more than about 10 minutes. The instructor will halt the role-play either at that time or when s/he feels that the scenario has been resolved.
3. For each role-play, the class should focus discussion on the following questions:
   a. In what ways, both verbally and nonverbally, was the response given in the scenario assertive, nonassertive, or aggressive?
   b. In what ways were both individuals' rights taken or not taken into account?
   c. What would be an aggressive response in the scenario, and why?
   d. What would be a nonassertive response in the scenario, and why?
   e. What would be the ideal way to resolve the situation assertively, and why?

Chapter 7 Competencies/Practice Behaviors Exercises Assessment:

Name: ______________________________ **Date:** __________
Supervisor's Name: ______________________

Focus Competencies/Practice Behaviors:

- EP 2.1.1b Practice personal reflection and self-correction to assure continual professional development
- EP 2.1.3c Demonstrate effective oral and written communication in working with individuals, families, groups, organizations, communities, and colleagues
- EP 2.1.4b Gain sufficient self-awareness to eliminate the influence of personal biases and values in working with diverse groups
- EP 2.1.4c Recognize and communicate their understanding of the importance of difference in shaping life experiences
- EP 2.1.7a Utilize conceptual frameworks to guide the processes of assessment, intervention, and evaluation
- EP 2.1.10a Substantively and affectively prepare for action with individuals, families, groups, organizations, and communities

Instructions:

A. Evaluate your work or your partner's work in the Focus Competencies/Practice Behaviors by completing the Competencies/Practice Behaviors Assessment form below

B. What other Competencies/Practice Behaviors did you use to complete these Exercises? Be sure to record them in your assessments

1.	I have attained this competency/practice behavior (in the range of 81 to 100%)
2.	I have largely attained this competency/practice behavior (in the range of 61 to 80%)
3.	I have partially attained this competency/practice behavior (in the range of 41 to 60%)
4.	I have made a little progress in attaining this competency/practice behavior (in the range of 21 to 40%)
5.	I have made almost no progress in attaining this competency/practice behavior (in the range of 0 to 20%)

EPAS 2008 Core Competencies & Core Practice Behaviors	Student Self Assessment						Evaluator Feedback
Student and Evaluator Assessment Scale and Comments	**0**	**1**	**2**	**3**	**4**	**5**	**Agree/Disagree/Comments**
EP 2.1.1 Identify as a Professional Social Worker and Conduct Oneself Accordingly:							
a. Advocate for client access to the services of social work							
b. Practice personal reflection and self-correction to assure continual professional development							
c. Attend to professional roles and boundaries							
d. Demonstrate professional demeanor in behavior, appearance, and communication							
e. Engage in career-long learning							
f. Use supervision and consultation							

EP 2.1.2 Apply Social Work Ethical Principles to Guide Professional Practice:							
a. Recognize and manage personal values in a way that allows professional values to guide practice							
b. Make ethical decisions by applying NASW Code of Ethics and, as applicable, of the IFSW/IASSW Ethics in Social Work, Statement of Principles							
c. Tolerate ambiguity in resolving ethical conflicts							
d. Apply strategies of ethical reasoning to arrive at principled decisions							
EP 2.1.3 Apply Critical Thinking to Inform and Communicate Professional Judgments:							
a. Distinguish, appraise, and integrate multiple sources of knowledge, including research-based knowledge and practice wisdom							
b. Analyze models of assessment, prevention, intervention, and evaluation							
c. Demonstrate effective oral and written communication in working with individuals, families, groups, organizations, communities, and colleagues							
EP 2.1.4 Engage Diversity and Difference in Practice:							
a. Recognize the extent to which a culture's structures and values may oppress, marginalize, alienate, or create or enhance privilege and power							
b. Gain sufficient self-awareness to eliminate the influence of personal biases and values in working with diverse groups							
c. Recognize and communicate their understanding of the importance of difference in shaping life experiences							
d. View themselves as learners and engage those with whom they work as informants							
EP 2.1.5 Advance Human Rights and Social and Economic Justice:							
a. Understand forms and mechanisms of oppression and discrimination							
b. Advocate for human rights and social and economic justice							
c. Engage in practices that advance social and economic justice							
EP 2.1.6 Engage in Research-Informed Practice and Practice-Informed Research:							
a. Use practice experience to inform scientific inquiry							
b. Use research evidence to inform practice							
EP 2.1.7 Apply Knowledge of Human Behavior and the Social Environment:							
a. Utilize conceptual frameworks to guide the processes of assessment, intervention, and evaluation							
b. Critique and apply knowledge to understand person and environment							

EP 2.1.8 Engage in Policy Practice to Advance Social and Economic Well-Being and to Deliver Effective Social Work Services:							
a. Analyze, formulate, and advocate for policies that advance social well-being							
b. Collaborate with colleagues and clients for effective policy action							
EP 2.1.9 Respond to Contexts that Shape Practice:							
a. Continuously discover, appraise, and attend to changing locales, populations, scientific and technological developments, and emerging societal trends to provide relevant services							
b. Provide leadership in promoting sustainable changes in service delivery and practice to improve the quality of social services							
EP 2.1.10 Engage, Assess, Intervene, and Evaluate with Individuals, Families, Groups, Organizations and Communities:							
a. Substantively and affectively prepare for action with individuals, families, groups, organizations, and communities							
b. Use empathy and other interpersonal skills							
c. Develop a mutually agreed-on focus of work and desired outcomes							
d. Collect, organize, and interpret client data							
e. Assess client strengths and limitations							
f. Develop mutually agreed-on intervention goals and objectives							
g. Select appropriate intervention strategies							
h. Initiate actions to achieve organizational goals							
i. Implement prevention interventions that enhance client capacities							
j. Help clients resolve problems							
k. Negotiate, mediate, and advocate for clients							
l. Facilitate transitions and endings							
m. Critically analyze, monitor, and evaluate interventions							

Chapter 8
Social Development in Adolescence

Competencies/Practice Behaviors Exercise 8.1
Changing Unwanted Emotions by Writing a Rational Self-Analysis

Focus Competencies or Practice Behaviors:

- EP 2.1.1b Practice personal reflection and self-correction to assure continual professional development
- EP 2.1.3b Analyze models of assessment, prevention, intervention, and evaluation
- EP 2.1.6b Use research evidence to inform practice
- EP 2.1.7a Utilize conceptual frameworks to guide the processes of assessment, intervention, and evaluation
- EP 2.1.7b Critique and apply knowledge to understand person and environment
- EP 2.1.10a Substantively and affectively prepare for action with individuals, families, groups, organizations, and communities
- EP 2.1.10j Help clients resolve problems
- EP 2.1.10m Critically analyze, monitor, and evaluate interventions

A. Brief description

You will write a rational self-analysis.

B. Objectives

You will:

1. Understand that unwanted emotions primarily result from negative and irrational thinking.
2. Change your unwanted emotions by challenging negative and irrational thinking with positive and rational self-talk.
3. Assist others in changing unwanted emotions by helping them to switch their negative and irrational self-talk to positive and rational self-talk.

C. Procedure

1. Summarize the material in the text that indicates that unwanted emotions are caused primarily by negative and irrational thinking.
2. The instructor describes how to write a rational self-analysis. Look at the example presented in the text.
3. Write a rational self-analysis of an unwanted emotion currently or recently experienced.
4. The instructor may ask for volunteers to share what they wrote.
5. What difficulties did you experience in writing a rational self-analysis? What did you see as the strengths and shortcomings of writing such an analysis?

Competencies/Practice Behaviors Exercise 8.2
Assessing and Treating Dysfunctional Behavior

Focus Competencies or Practice Behaviors:

- EP 2.1.1b Practice personal reflection and self-correction to assure continual professional development
- EP 2.1.3b Analyze models of assessment, prevention, intervention, and evaluation
- EP 2.1.7a Utilize conceptual frameworks to guide the processes of assessment, intervention, and evaluation
- EP 2.1.7b Critique and apply knowledge to understand person and environment
- EP 2.1.10a Substantively and affectively prepare for action with individuals, families, groups, organizations, and communities
- EP 2.1.10j Help clients resolve problems
- EP 2.1.10m Critically analyze, monitor, and evaluate interventions

A. Brief description

You will assess dysfunctional behavior by identifying underlying thinking patterns of the perpetrators and then discuss various treatment approaches for changing these underlying thinking patterns.

B. Objectives

You will:

1. Understand the principle that thinking processes primarily determine behavior, including dysfunctional behavior.
2. Apply the rational therapy approach to assessing and treating dysfunctional behavior.

C. Procedure

1. The instructor summarizes the material on rational therapy in the text, which asserts that the reasons for dysfunctional behavior occurring can be identified by determining what the perpetrator was thinking.
2. Divide into subgroups of about five persons. Each subgroup is given a card that has one of the following dysfunctional behaviors written on it: compulsive gambling, date rape, prostitution, suicide, alcoholism, anorexic behavior, bulimic behavior, child abuse, and wife abuse. Each subgroup receives a different dysfunctional behavior and tries to identify the thinking processes that would lead a person to engage in this behavior.
3. Identify the interventions that you believe would be most effective in changing the thinking patterns of a person with this problematic behavior so that the person would be unlikely to continue engaging in such dysfunctional behavior.
4. Each subgroup reports to the class on the thinking patterns of the dysfunctional behavior and the intervention approaches it identified. After each subgroup makes its presentation, the rest of the class is given an opportunity to add to the information being reported by the subgroup.
5. Discuss the merits and shortcomings of assessing behavior by identifying the thinking patterns of the perpetrator.

Competencies/Practice Behaviors Exercise 8.3
Mental Illness Debate Role-Play

Focus Competencies or Practice Behaviors:

- EP 2.1.1b Practice personal reflection and self-correction to assure continual professional development
- EP 2.1.3a Distinguish, appraise, and integrate multiple sources of knowledge, including research-based knowledge and practice wisdom
- EP 2.1.3b Analyze models of assessment, prevention, intervention, and evaluation
- EP 2.1.6b Use research evidence to inform practice
- EP 2.1.7a Utilize conceptual frameworks to guide the processes of assessment, intervention, and evaluation
- EP 2.1.7b Critique and apply knowledge to understand person and environment

A. Brief description

A debate will be held in class about whether or not mental illness exists.

B. Objectives

You will:

1. Understand the arguments regarding whether mental illness exists.
2. Understand the effects of labeling someone "mentally ill."

C. Procedure

1. Read the material in the chapter related to the medical model approach and the interactional model approach to emotional and behavioral problems. At a class session, select some students to form two panels, one to argue that mental illness exists and the other that it is a myth. Panel members should be given a few days to gather additional information to prepare for a debate. Panel members may choose to interview counselors and therapists in the community. Panel members should definitely read reference material related to this topic; the instructor may serve as a resource for such material.
2. On a day selected by the class, a debate is held. At the end of the debate, the students who were not involved in the debate summarize the strong points made by the debaters.

Competencies/Practice Behaviors Exercise 8.4
Trust Walk

Focus Competencies or Practice Behaviors:

- EP 2.1.1b Practice personal reflection and self-correction to assure continual professional development

A. Brief description

You and other students in class become involved in trust walks.

B. Objectives

You will:

1. Learn how to conduct a trust walk.
2. Get in touch with aspects of yourself that you are unaware of.

C. Procedure

1. The instructor informs the class of the objectives of the exercise. The instructor has the students form groups of two. (If a student is without a partner, the instructor can be a partner.)
2. One member of your subgroup closes his or her eyes, and keeps the eyes closed for the first part of this exercise. The "seeing" partner then leads the "blind" partner down corridors, around the room, and perhaps outside. The "seeing" partner can lead the "blind" partner with verbal directions and by taking a hand. The "seeing" person has the responsibility to watch that the "blind" partner does not run into objects, fall, stumble, or get hurt in any way.
3. After 8 to 10 minutes, the partners reverse roles and continue the exercise for another 8 to 10 minutes.
4. You and other students, as a class, then discuss the feelings experienced while doing this trust walk.

Chapter 8 Competencies/Practice Behaviors Exercises Assessment:

Name: ____ **Date:** ____________
Supervisor's Name: ____________________________

Focus Competencies or Practice Behaviors:

- EP 2.1.1b Practice personal reflection and self-correction to assure continual professional development
- EP 2.1.3a Distinguish, appraise, and integrate multiple sources of knowledge, including research-based knowledge and practice wisdom
- EP 2.1.3b Analyze models of assessment, prevention, intervention, and evaluation
- EP 2.1.6b Use research evidence to inform practice
- EP 2.1.7a Utilize conceptual frameworks to guide the processes of assessment, intervention, and evaluation
- EP 2.1.7b Critique and apply knowledge to understand person and environment
- EP 2.1.10a Substantively and affectively prepare for action with individuals, families, groups, organizations, and communities
- EP 2.1.10j Help clients resolve problems
- EP 2.1.10m Critically analyze, monitor, and evaluate interventions

Instructions:

A. Evaluate your work or your partner's work in the Focus Competencies/Practice Behaviors by completing the Competencies/Practice Behaviors Assessment form below

B. What other Competencies/Practice Behaviors did you use to complete these Exercises? Be sure to record them in your assessments

1.	I have attained this competency/practice behavior (in the range of 81 to 100%)
2.	I have largely attained this competency/practice behavior (in the range of 61 to 80%)
3.	I have partially attained this competency/practice behavior (in the range of 41 to 60%)
4.	I have made a little progress in attaining this competency/practice behavior (in the range of 21 to 40%)
5.	I have made almost no progress in attaining this competency/practice behavior (in the range of 0 to 20%)

EPAS 2008 Core Competencies & Core Practice Behaviors	**Student Self Assessment**						**Evaluator Feedback**
Student and Evaluator Assessment Scale and Comments	**0**	**1**	**2**	**3**	**4**	**5**	**Agree/Disagree/Comments**
EP 2.1.1 Identify as a Professional Social Worker and Conduct Oneself Accordingly:							
a. Advocate for client access to the services of social work							
b. Practice personal reflection and self-correction to assure continual professional development							
c. Attend to professional roles and boundaries							
d. Demonstrate professional demeanor in behavior, appearance, and communication							
e. Engage in career-long learning							
f. Use supervision and consultation							

EP 2.1.2 Apply Social Work Ethical Principles to Guide Professional Practice:							
a. Recognize and manage personal values in a way that allows professional values to guide practice							
b. Make ethical decisions by applying NASW Code of Ethics and, as applicable, of the IFSW/IASSW Ethics in Social Work, Statement of Principles							
c. Tolerate ambiguity in resolving ethical conflicts							
d. Apply strategies of ethical reasoning to arrive at principled decisions							
EP 2.1.3 Apply Critical Thinking to Inform and Communicate Professional Judgments:							
a. Distinguish, appraise, and integrate multiple sources of knowledge, including research-based knowledge and practice wisdom							
b. Analyze models of assessment, prevention, intervention, and evaluation							
c. Demonstrate effective oral and written communication in working with individuals, families, groups, organizations, communities, and colleagues							
EP 2.1.4 Engage Diversity and Difference in Practice:							
a. Recognize the extent to which a culture's structures and values may oppress, marginalize, alienate, or create or enhance privilege and power							
b. Gain sufficient self-awareness to eliminate the influence of personal biases and values in working with diverse groups							
c. Recognize and communicate their understanding of the importance of difference in shaping life experiences							
d. View themselves as learners and engage those with whom they work as informants							
EP 2.1.5 Advance Human Rights and Social and Economic Justice:							
a. Understand forms and mechanisms of oppression and discrimination							
b. Advocate for human rights and social and economic justice							
c. Engage in practices that advance social and economic justice							
EP 2.1.6 Engage in Research-Informed Practice and Practice-Informed Research:							
a. Use practice experience to inform scientific inquiry							
b. Use research evidence to inform practice							
EP 2.1.7 Apply Knowledge of Human Behavior and the Social Environment:							
a. Utilize conceptual frameworks to guide the processes of assessment, intervention, and evaluation							
b. Critique and apply knowledge to understand person and environment							

EP 2.1.8 Engage in Policy Practice to Advance Social and Economic Well-Being and to Deliver Effective Social Work Services:							
a. Analyze, formulate, and advocate for policies that advance social well-being							
b. Collaborate with colleagues and clients for effective policy action							
EP 2.1.9 Respond to Contexts that Shape Practice:							
a. Continuously discover, appraise, and attend to changing locales, populations, scientific and technological developments, and emerging societal trends to provide relevant services							
b. Provide leadership in promoting sustainable changes in service delivery and practice to improve the quality of social services							
EP 2.1.10 Engage, Assess, Intervene, and Evaluate with Individuals, Families, Groups, Organizations and Communities:							
a. Substantively and affectively prepare for action with individuals, families, groups, organizations, and communities							
b. Use empathy and other interpersonal skills							
c. Develop a mutually agreed-on focus of work and desired outcomes							
d. Collect, organize, and interpret client data							
e. Assess client strengths and limitations							
f. Develop mutually agreed-on intervention goals and objectives							
g. Select appropriate intervention strategies							
h. Initiate actions to achieve organizational goals							
i. Implement prevention interventions that enhance client capacities							
j. Help clients resolve problems							
k. Negotiate, mediate, and advocate for clients							
l. Facilitate transitions and endings							
m. Critically analyze, monitor, and evaluate interventions							

Chapter 9
Gender, Gender Identity, Gender Expression, and Sexism

Competencies/Practice Behaviors Exercise 9.1
Media Craze

Focus Competencies or Practice Behaviors:

- EP 2.1.1b Practice personal reflection and self-correction to assure continual professional development
- EP 2.1.2a Recognize and manage personal values in a way that allows professional values to guide practice
- EP 2.1.4a Recognize the extent to which a culture's structures and values may oppress, marginalize, alienate, or create or enhance privilege and power
- EP 2.1.4b Gain sufficient self-awareness to eliminate the influence of personal biases and values in working with diverse groups
- EP 2.1.4c Recognize and communicate their understanding of the importance of difference in shaping life experiences
- EP 2.1.5a Understand forms and mechanisms of oppression and discrimination
- EP 2.1.7b Critique and apply knowledge to understand person and environment

A. Brief description
You are shown various magazine advertisements, and are asked to discuss how gender roles and sexist ideas are portrayed by the pictures.

B. Objectives
You will:
1. Identify how the media depict men and women.
2. Examine common sexist biases.
3. Propose alternative, nonsexist approaches to advertising.

C. Procedure
1. While looking at each picture, discuss the following questions:
    a. What does this picture convey about how women and men are or should be?
    b. What are your reactions as to how these attitudes relate to you?
    c. How might the product be portrayed in a nonsexist manner?

Competencies/Practice Behaviors Exercise 9.2
Have Things Really Changed Role-Play

Focus Competencies or Practice Behaviors:

- EP 2.1.1b Practice personal reflection and self-correction to assure continual professional development
- EP 2.1.2a Recognize and manage personal values in a way that allows professional values to guide practice
- EP 2.1.4a Recognize the extent to which a culture's structures and values may oppress, marginalize, alienate, or create or enhance privilege and power

- EP 2.1.4b Gain sufficient self-awareness to eliminate the influence of personal biases and values in working with diverse groups
- EP 2.1.4c Recognize and communicate their understanding of the importance of difference in shaping life experiences
- EP 2.1.5a Understand forms and mechanisms of oppression and discrimination
- EP 2.1.5b Advocate for human rights and social and economic justice
- EP 2.1.7b Critique and apply knowledge to understand person and environment

A. Brief description

You will discuss specific questions about current gender role expectations.

B. Objectives

You will:

1. Examine some issues concerning the equality or lack of equality of gender roles.
2. Evaluate some current gender role expectations.
3. Propose suggestions for correcting discrepancies between the gender roles that you judge to be unfair.

C. Procedure

1. Divide into groups of four to six persons.
2. Discuss each of the following questions, one question at a time:
   a. Should women ask men for dates?
   b. Is there still a double standard concerning premarital sex?
   c. Should mothers work outside the home or try to stay home with their young children?
3. You have approximately 10 minutes to discuss each question. After each question, a volunteer from each group summarizes its conclusions for the class, and a short discussion follows.
4. After addressing each question, the entire class addresses the following questions:
   a. Are there any differences between how you think things should be and what you would actually do yourself if involved in situations similar to those discussed?
   b. In regard to the situations you discussed in small groups, to what extent do you think things have changed from the traditional ways?
   c. What things might be done to increase the equality between men and women?

Competencies/Practice Behaviors Exercise 9.3
Girls Are This Way, Boys Are That Way

Focus Competencies or Practice Behaviors:

- EP 2.1.1b Practice personal reflection and self-correction to assure continual professional development
- EP 2.1.2a Recognize and manage personal values in a way that allows professional values to guide practice
- EP 2.1.4a Recognize the extent to which a culture's structures and values may oppress, marginalize, alienate, or create or enhance privilege and power
- EP 2.1.4b Gain sufficient self-awareness to eliminate the influence of personal biases and values in working with diverse groups

- EP 2.1.4c Recognize and communicate their understanding of the importance of difference in shaping life experiences
- EP 2.1.5a Understand forms and mechanisms of oppression and discrimination
- EP 2.1.7b Critique and apply knowledge to understand person and environment

A. Brief description

You will examine and discuss how traditional gender-role stereotypes characterize both females and males and evaluate the effects of these stereotypes.

B. Objectives

You will:

1. Identify stereotypes and characteristics traditionally associated with the respective gender roles.
2. Appraise the effects of these stereotypes on people's right to individuality.

C. Procedure

1. As an introduction to lecturing about and discussing sexism, the instructor will write the following open-ended statements on the board:
   Females are ___.
   Males are ___.
2. Call out some of the characteristics that males and females traditionally are supposed to have. The instructor writes the responses on the board.
3. Discuss the following questions:
   a. To what extent do these stereotypes apply to people's behavior today?
   b. How do these stereotypes affect people's right to individuality—the right to be themselves without uncomfortable pretense?

Competencies/Practice Behaviors Exercise 9.4
The Fishbowl

Focus Competencies or Practice Behaviors:

- EP 2.1.2a Recognize and manage personal values in a way that allows professional values to guide practice
- EP 2.1.4c Recognize and communicate their understanding of the importance of difference in shaping life experiences
- EP 2.1.5a Understand forms and mechanisms of oppression and discrimination
- EP 2.1.7b Critique and apply knowledge to understand person and environment

A. Brief description

You will form two groups according to gender and discuss various aspects you find attractive in the opposite gender. Discussion will follow regarding the perceptions.

B. Objectives

You will:

1. Describe your feelings regarding positive qualities of the opposite gender.
2. Examine some of your misconceptions about the opposite gender.
3. Assess similarities and differences in the perceptions of each gender.

C. Procedure

1. Form two groups, one including all the females and the other all the males.
2. The females sit in an inner circle in the center of the classroom. The males position themselves in an outer circle around the females.
3. The females discuss what **physical, emotional, and behavioral** characteristics they find attractive in males. The males remain silent. The discussion continues for 10 to 15 minutes.
4. Reverse positions; males should sit in the inner circle and females in the outer one. The males discuss what **physical, emotional, and behavioral** characteristics they find attractive in females. This time, the females remain silent.
5. You will have 10 to 15 minutes of discussion. Then the entire class discusses the following questions:
   a. What did you learn about the opposite gender from this exercise?
   b. Were there any surprises?
   c. What were some of the similarities and some of the differences between females' and males' perceptions?

Competencies/Practice Behaviors Exercise 9.5
Life Questions

Focus Competencies or Practice Behaviors:

- EP 2.1.1b Practice personal reflection and self-correction to assure continual professional development
- EP 2.1.2a Recognize and manage personal values in a way that allows professional values to guide practice
- EP 2.1.4a Recognize the extent to which a culture's structures and values may oppress, marginalize, alienate, or create or enhance privilege and power
- EP 2.1.4b Gain sufficient self-awareness to eliminate the influence of personal biases and values in working with diverse groups
- EP 2.1.4c Recognize and communicate their understanding of the importance of difference in shaping life experiences
- EP 2.1.5a Understand forms and mechanisms of oppression and discrimination
- EP 2.1.5b Advocate for human rights and social and economic justice
- EP 2.1.7a Utilize conceptual frameworks to guide the processes of assessment, intervention, and evaluation

A. Brief description

You will be given a variety of thought-provoking questions concerning male and female gender roles and asked to discuss your own opinions.

B. Objectives

You will:

1. Recognize your personal opinions and biases on a number of gender issues including treatment on the job, leadership, pregnancy, and household tasks.
2. Examine the distribution of power and opportunity between genders on these issues and assess the extent to which the situations are fair.
3. Formulate suggestions for addressing these issues.

C. Procedure

1. Form small groups of four to six persons.
2. Discuss the following questions. Write down your opinions on the question sheet. At the end of the exercise, a volunteer from each group will summarize your findings and ideas for the entire class.

LIFE QUESTIONS

1. Treatment on the Job

   a. Should men and women be treated equally on the job?

2. Leadership

   a. When you get a job, would you prefer a man or a woman as a supervisor?

   b. What are the reasons for your answer?

3. Pregnancy

   a. Should a working woman be granted a leave of absence for pregnancy?

   b. Why or why not?

   c. If so, for how long?

   d. Should the leave be with or without pay?

   e. Do you think mothers of young children should stay home to take care of them?

   f. Should fathers of newborn infants be given leaves of absence? If so, this should occur under what circumstances (e.g., length of time, paid or unpaid)?

4. Household Tasks

a. Do married men and women share household tasks equally these days (for example, taking out the garbage, cleaning the bathroom, doing the laundry, washing dishes, cooking, grocery shopping, taking care of the kids)?

b. Do you think household tasks should be shared equally by a male and female living together as spouses or partners?

c. If you marry (or are married), do you plan to share household tasks equally? Explain why or why not.

3. A volunteer from your group should summarize your findings for the entire class. The class then addresses the following questions:
   a. Are power and opportunity distributed fairly between genders? Why or why not?
   b. What are your opinions and biases about these issues? How do these coincide with professional social work values?
   c. In those instances where you perceive inequities, what changes should be made?

Chapter 9 Competencies/Practice Behaviors Exercises Assessment:

Name: ______________________ **Date:** ____________
Supervisor's Name: ______________________

Focus Competencies or Practice Behaviors:

- EP 2.1.1b Practice personal reflection and self-correction to assure continual professional development
- EP 2.1.2a Recognize and manage personal values in a way that allows professional values to guide practice
- EP 2.1.4a Recognize the extent to which a culture's structures and values may oppress, marginalize, alienate, or create or enhance privilege and power
- EP 2.1.4b Gain sufficient self-awareness to eliminate the influence of personal biases and values in working with diverse groups
- EP 2.1.4c Recognize and communicate their understanding of the importance of difference in shaping life experiences
- EP 2.1.5a Understand forms and mechanisms of oppression and discrimination
- EP 2.1.5b Advocate for human rights and social and economic justice
- EP 2.1.7a Utilize conceptual frameworks to guide the processes of assessment, intervention, and evaluation
- EP 2.1.7b Critique and apply knowledge to understand person and environment

Instructions:

A. Evaluate your work or your partner's work in the Focus Competencies/Practice Behaviors by completing the Competencies/Practice Behaviors Assessment form below

B. What other Competencies/Practice Behaviors did you use to complete these Exercises? Be sure to record them in your assessments

1.	I have attained this competency/practice behavior (in the range of 81 to 100%)
2.	I have largely attained this competency/practice behavior (in the range of 61 to 80%)
3.	I have partially attained this competency/practice behavior (in the range of 41 to 60%)
4.	I have made a little progress in attaining this competency/practice behavior (in the range of 21 to 40%)
5.	I have made almost no progress in attaining this competency/practice behavior (in the range of 0 to 20%)

EPAS 2008 Core Competencies & Core Practice Behaviors	Student Self Assessment						Evaluator Feedback
Student and Evaluator Assessment Scale and Comments	**0**	**1**	**2**	**3**	**4**	**5**	**Agree/Disagree/Comments**
EP 2.1.1 Identify as a Professional Social Worker and Conduct Oneself Accordingly:							
a. Advocate for client access to the services of social work							
b. Practice personal reflection and self-correction to assure continual professional development							
c. Attend to professional roles and boundaries							
d. Demonstrate professional demeanor in behavior, appearance, and communication							
e. Engage in career-long learning							
f. Use supervision and consultation							

EP 2.1.2 Apply Social Work Ethical Principles to Guide Professional Practice:								
a.	Recognize and manage personal values in a way that allows professional values to guide practice							
b.	Make ethical decisions by applying NASW Code of Ethics and, as applicable, of the IFSW/IASSW Ethics in Social Work, Statement of Principles							
c.	Tolerate ambiguity in resolving ethical conflicts							
d.	Apply strategies of ethical reasoning to arrive at principled decisions							
EP 2.1.3 Apply Critical Thinking to Inform and Communicate Professional Judgments:								
a.	Distinguish, appraise, and integrate multiple sources of knowledge, including research-based knowledge and practice wisdom							
b.	Analyze models of assessment, prevention, intervention, and evaluation							
c.	Demonstrate effective oral and written communication in working with individuals, families, groups, organizations, communities, and colleagues							
EP 2.1.4 Engage Diversity and Difference in Practice:								
a.	Recognize the extent to which a culture's structures and values may oppress, marginalize, alienate, or create or enhance privilege and power							
b.	Gain sufficient self-awareness to eliminate the influence of personal biases and values in working with diverse groups							
c.	Recognize and communicate their understanding of the importance of difference in shaping life experiences							
d.	View themselves as learners and engage those with whom they work as informants							
EP 2.1.5 Advance Human Rights and Social and Economic Justice:								
a.	Understand forms and mechanisms of oppression and discrimination							
b.	Advocate for human rights and social and economic justice							
c.	Engage in practices that advance social and economic justice							
EP 2.1.6 Engage in Research-Informed Practice and Practice-Informed Research:								
a.	Use practice experience to inform scientific inquiry							
b.	Use research evidence to inform practice							
EP 2.1.7 Apply Knowledge of Human Behavior and the Social Environment:								
a.	Utilize conceptual frameworks to guide the processes of assessment, intervention, and evaluation							
b.	Critique and apply knowledge to understand person and environment							

EP 2.1.8 Engage in Policy Practice to Advance Social and Economic Well-Being and to Deliver Effective Social Work Services:							
a. Analyze, formulate, and advocate for policies that advance social well-being							
b. Collaborate with colleagues and clients for effective policy action							
EP 2.1.9 Respond to Contexts that Shape Practice:							
a. Continuously discover, appraise, and attend to changing locales, populations, scientific and technological developments, and emerging societal trends to provide relevant services							
b. Provide leadership in promoting sustainable changes in service delivery and practice to improve the quality of social services							
EP 2.1.10 Engage, Assess, Intervene, and Evaluate with Individuals, Families, Groups, Organizations and Communities:							
a. Substantively and affectively prepare for action with individuals, families, groups, organizations, and communities							
b. Use empathy and other interpersonal skills							
c. Develop a mutually agreed-on focus of work and desired outcomes							
d. Collect, organize, and interpret client data							
e. Assess client strengths and limitations							
f. Develop mutually agreed-on intervention goals and objectives							
g. Select appropriate intervention strategies							
h. Initiate actions to achieve organizational goals							
i. Implement prevention interventions that enhance client capacities							
j. Help clients resolve problems							
k. Negotiate, mediate, and advocate for clients							
l. Facilitate transitions and endings							
m. Critically analyze, monitor, and evaluate interventions							

Chapter 10
Biological Aspects of Young and Middle Adulthood

Competencies/Practice Behaviors Exercise 10.1
To Be Healthy or Not To Be Healthy: That Is the Question

Focus Competencies or Practice Behaviors:

- EP 2.1.1b Practice personal reflection and self-correction to assure continual professional development
- EP 2.1.3a Distinguish, appraise, and integrate multiple sources of knowledge, including research-based knowledge and practice wisdom
- EP 2.1.3b Analyze models of assessment, prevention, intervention, and evaluation
- EP 2.1.7a Utilize conceptual frameworks to guide the processes of assessment, intervention, and evaluation
- EP 2.1.7b Critique and apply knowledge to understand person and environment
- EP 2.1.10a Substantively and affectively prepare for action with individuals, families, groups, organizations, and communities

A. Brief description

Aspects of your own healthful behavior are examined. In small groups you will discuss how unhealthful behaviors are maintained and address the difficulties involved in changing poor health behaviors.

B. Objectives

You will:

1. Identify some of the lifestyle habits that contribute to good health and some that are hazardous to health.
2. Examine the advantages and disadvantages of various poor health habits.
3. Propose how the behaviors that are related to poor health might be changed.
4. Assess the difficulties involved in changing poor health habits.
5. Relate these difficulties to the difficulties clients have in changing their lifestyle habits.

C. Procedure

1. Review the material in the text that addresses lifestyle and good health.
2. Place a check mark before any of the following poor health habits that you feel are a regular part of your lifestyle.

Do you:

_____ rarely if ever eat breakfast
_____ rarely if ever eat regular meals
_____ frequently snack between meals
_____ smoke cigarettes regularly
_____ rarely if ever participate in moderate physical exercise
_____ get less than 7 to 8 hours sleep each night on a regular basis
_____ drink alcoholic beverages frequently and in large quantities

3. Break into groups of four to six persons. Discuss the following questions:
   a. Why do people participate in each of the listed behaviors?
   b. What are the advantages or benefits for them?
   c. What are the disadvantages for people who participate in each of these behaviors?
   d. How might people go about changing unhealthful habits and behaviors?
   e. What are the difficulties involved in trying to change each of these behaviors?
4. You will have approximately 20 minutes for discussion. All group members are encouraged to participate. You need not divulge any of your personal habits if you don't choose to.
5. After 20 minutes all small groups join in a summary discussion. Choose a representative from your group to summarize information discussed by your group. Each group should report on one of the seven bad habits. Your representative should summarize the group's discussion concerning all five of the questions in relationship to one poor health habit.
6. Summarize the difficulties in changing poor health habits. Relate this to how difficult it is for clients to change their life-style habits and behaviors.

Competencies/Practice Behaviors Exercise 10.2
Extramarital Affairs

Focus Competencies or Practice Behaviors:

- EP 2.1.1b Practice personal reflection and self-correction to assure continual professional development

A. Brief description

This is a values-clarification exercise about issues relating to extramarital sexual relationships.

B. Objectives

You will:

1. State your values about extramarital affairs and mate-swapping arrangements.

C. Procedures

1. Form subgroups of about five persons and seek a group consensus about the following questions (the questions should be written on the board).
   a. Do you think extramarital affairs are ever justified (for example, when one's spouse is physically unable to have sex)? If yes, in what circumstances are they justified?
   b. If you were married, would you want to participate in a mate-swapping arrangement? Why or why not?
2. After you have arrived at answers, a representative from each subgroup shares the views of the subgroup.

Competencies/Practice Behaviors Exercise 10.3
AIDS and Values Clarification

Focus Competencies or Practice Behaviors:

- EP 2.1.1b Practice personal reflection and self-correction to assure continual professional development
- EP 2.1.2a Recognize and manage personal values in a way that allows professional values to guide practice
- EP 2.1.2b Make ethical decisions by applying standards of the National Association of Social Workers Code of Ethics and, as applicable, of the International Federation of Social Workers/International Association of Schools of Social Work Ethics in Social Work, Statement of Principles
- EP 2.1.3a Distinguish, appraise, and integrate multiple sources of knowledge, including research-based knowledge and practice wisdom
- EP 2.1.6b Use research evidence to inform practice
- EP 2.1.7a Utilize conceptual frameworks to guide the processes of assessment, intervention, and evaluation

A. Brief description
You will fill out a values-clarification questionnaire on issues related to AIDS.

B. Objectives
You will:
1. State your values about issues related to AIDS.
2. Receive information that will enable you to be more objective about AIDS.

C. Procedure
1. On a separate sheet of paper anonymously mark your answers to the following questions:

AIDS QUESTIONNAIRE

1. Would you be comfortable working in the same office with another employee that is known to be infected with HIV?
____ Yes ____ Uncertain ____ No

2. If you were a parent, would you send your child to a school in which a classmate is known to be infected with HIV?
____ Yes ____ Uncertain ____ No

3. Assume you are a social worker in a nursing home. Would you be comfortable working with residents who have AIDS?
____ Yes ____ Uncertain ____ No

4. Would you feel comfortable in hugging someone who has AIDS?
____ Yes ____ Uncertain ____ No

5. Do you believe that the peril of AIDS is a punishment from a higher being for homosexual behavior?
____ Yes ____ Uncertain ____ No

6. If you were a parent, would you be comfortable seeing your children play with a neighborhood child who has tested positive for HIV?
____ Yes ____ Uncertain ____ No

7. Would you feel comfortable living with a roommate who has HIV?
____ Yes ____ Uncertain ____ No

8. Do you believe AIDS can be transmitted by mosquito bites?
____ Yes ____ Uncertain ____ No

9. Would you hesitate to swim in a swimming pool in which someone else is swimming who you know has HIV?
____ Yes ____ Uncertain ____ No

10. Do you believe people should restrict their sexual activity to safe (safer) sex practices?
____ Yes ____ Uncertain ____ No

11. If you discovered that someone you were dating tested positive for HIV, would you seek to terminate the relationship?
____ Yes ____ Uncertain ____ No

12. If you tested positive for HIV, would you contemplate suicide?
____ Yes ____ Uncertain ____ No

13. If you discover your physician or dentist is HIV positive, would you discontinue receiving services from this physician or dentist?
____ Yes ____ Uncertain ____ No

2. While you are recording your answers, the instructor lists the 13 question numbers on the chalkboard according to the following format:

	Yes	Uncertain	No
1.			
2.			
3.			
etc.			

3. Anonymously hand in your answers. Volunteers will list the students' responses on the chalkboard.
4. The instructor reads each question out loud and then reviews student answers. The instructor may want to present objective information as these questions are being reviewed. Share your thoughts and feelings and ask any questions you have.

Competencies/Practice Behaviors Exercise 10.4
AIDS Policy Quiz

Focus Competencies or Practice Behaviors:

- EP 2.1.1b Practice personal reflection and self-correction to assure continual professional development
- EP 2.1.2a Recognize and manage personal values in a way that allows professional values to guide practice
- EP 2.1.2b Make ethical decisions by applying standards of the National Association of Social Workers Code of Ethics and, as applicable, of the International Federation of Social Workers/International Association of Schools of Social Work Ethics in Social Work, Statement of Principles
- EP 2.1.3a Distinguish, appraise, and integrate multiple sources of knowledge, including research-based knowledge and practice wisdom
- EP 2.1.6b Use research evidence to inform practice
- EP 2.1.7a Utilize conceptual frameworks to guide the processes of assessment, intervention, and evaluation
- EP 2.1.7b Critique and apply knowledge to understand person and environment

A. Brief description

You will take an AIDS POLICY QUIZ, which forces you to confront some of the complicated and difficult policy choices concerning AIDS.

B. Objectives

You will:

1. Recognize some of the disturbing and complex social policy issues involved in the AIDS epidemic.
2. Examine your own values and opinions about AIDS and persons living with AIDS.
3. Identify some of the issues facing persons with AIDS.

C. Procedure

1. The instructor reads aloud the following questions. As the instructor reads each question, you should read along in this workbook. After each question, the instructor asks for a show of hands indicating "yes" and "no" responses.

AIDS POLICY QUIZ

		Yes	No
1.	Should testing for HIV antibodies be made mandatory for hospital patients?	___	___
2.	Should the patient be required to pay for such testing?	___	___
3.	Should private insurance companies be required to pay for such testing for insured patients?	___	___
4.	If no other funding is available, should hospitals be required to pay for testing?	___	___

5. Should physicians and other health care workers be required to treat HIV positive patients? ___ ___

6. If you had a cancerous brain tumor, would you want a physician to be forced to do the surgery against his or her will? ___ ___

7. Should all people be required to have HIV testing before they get married? ___ ___

8. Should all students at your college or university be required to get HIV testing as part of their entrance physical exam? ___ ___

9. Should students be required to pay for the testing as part of their fees? ___ ___

10. Should students who test positive be denied admission to your college or university? ___ ___

11. Should all HIV testing be anonymous? ___ ___

12. Should positive results, along with the names of the persons who test positive, be reported to a state agency? ___ ___

13. Should these results and the names of persons testing positive be available to the public? ___ ___

14. Should people who test positive be required to submit the names of sexual partners to a state agency? ___ ___

15. Should these sexual partners be notified? ___ ___

16. Should these sexual partners be required to have HIV tests? ___ ___

17. Should positive results for sexual partners, along with the names of these persons, be reported to a state agency? ___ ___

18. Should the sexual partners of persons testing positive be required to pay for their own testing? ___ ___

19. Should employers be given the names of persons testing HIV positive? ___ ___

20. Should employers be allowed to dismiss persons testing HIV positive? ___ ___

21. Should insurance companies be alerted when someone covered by their policies is tested HIV positive? ___ ___

22. Should insurance companies be allowed to drop coverage of persons testing HIV positive in view of the tremendous expenses likely to be incurred? ___ ___

23.	Should insurance companies be given the option of denying coverage to those who have tested HIV positive just as they can deny coverage to those with prior conditions such as heart problems or back injuries?	___	___
24.	Should all insurance premiums be raised, taking money from all participants in the program, in order to cover the additional health expenses incurred by people with AIDS?	___	___
25.	Should people who know they test HIV positive and who have unprotected sexual relations or share IV drug needles with others without telling them that they're HIV positive be legally prosecuted?	___	___
26.	Should health care workers (such as physicians, dentists, and nurses) who test HIV positive be required to inform their patients of the results?	___	___
27.	Should all health care workers receive mandatory HIV testing?	___	___
28.	Should surgeons who test HIV positive be allowed to continue to perform surgery?	___	___
29.	If you discover your physician is HIV positive, would you discontinue receiving services from her or him?	___	___
30.	If you discover your dentist is HIV positive, would you discontinue receiving services from her or him?	___	___
31.	Assume you are a social worker for a client who reveals he just discovered he is HIV infected. The client refuses to inform his sexual partner of his HIV infection, for fear that the partner will end the sexual relationship. Would you break confidentiality and inform the sexual partner that the client has tested positive for HIV?	___	___
32.	Should free needles be distributed to intravenous drug users in an effort to reduce sharing of contaminated needles among IV drug users?	___	___
33.	Should condoms be distributed at no charge to adolescents at school in an effort to prevent the spread of HIV?	___	___
34.	Should surgeons be allowed to require that patients be tested for HIV prior to having surgery?	___	___
35.	Should all pregnant women be required to be tested for HIV, as there now is a treatment regimen (if started early in pregnancy) that reduces the chances that the child will be born infected with HIV?	___	___
36.	Should people testing HIV positive be required to wear an emblem in clear view at all times signifying that they are HIV positive?	___	___

2. After you've finished the quiz, discuss your feelings and reactions to taking it. You might focus on the following questions:
   a. How did you feel about the questions on the quiz?
   b. Which questions and policy issues concerned you the most?
   c. What do you think are possible solutions to these questions?
   d. What will the costs be for solutions?
   e. What would you be willing to sacrifice financially to attain these solutions?
   f. As a social worker, how might you function as an advocate for persons with AIDS?

Competencies/Practice Behaviors Exercise 10.5
Persons Living With AIDS Role-Play

Focus Competencies or Practice Behaviors:

- EP 2.1.1b Practice personal reflection and self-correction to assure continual professional development
- EP 2.1.3a Distinguish, appraise, and integrate multiple sources of knowledge, including research-based knowledge and practice wisdom
- EP 2.1.6b Use research evidence to inform practice
- EP 2.1.7b Critique and apply knowledge to understand person and environment
- EP 2.1.10a Substantively and affectively prepare for action with individuals, families, groups, organizations, and communities

A. Brief description
Vignettes concerning persons living with AIDS are presented, and you are asked to role-play how a social worker might help these persons.

B. Objectives
You will:
1. Formulate plans to empower persons with AIDS in a variety of situations.
2. Propose laws and social policies that would be helpful to persons with AIDS.

C. Procedure
1. Review the concept of empowerment and then role-play the following series of vignettes that illustrate a variety of situations involving people with AIDS. After each vignette, answer the following questions:
   a. In what ways could empowerment take place?
   b. In what ways could a social worker be helpful in this situation?
   c. What laws and social policies would be helpful to the AIDS sufferers in their situations?

PERSONS WITH AIDS

A. Mary has AIDS. She's 38 and used to have a lucrative law practice. She had been dating Norm and having intercourse with him for a year and a half before he told her that he was bisexual, that he had tested positively for HIV antibodies, and that she had better get tested, too. She dropped him immediately. The first time she had a test, the results were negative. However, the physician told her to come in once again in three months just to be sure. The second time she tested positive. Her rage was almost uncontrollable. It wasn't fair! She didn't "sleep around!" She didn't use intravenous drugs! Now Mary rarely leaves her apartment. She's terrified of being vulnerable to the multitude of diseases running rampant among all of the people out there. She knows that people are much more dangerous to her than she is to them. She desperately feels she needs to isolate herself. Her savings are dwindling. She can't afford to worry about the future.

B. Harry has been diagnosed positive for HIV antibodies in his system. Harry is only 22 and likes to party. He can hardly remember how many women he's had sexual intercourse with over the past two years. He's tall and handsome. Women have found him attractive as long as he can remember. He's always left the birth control responsibility up to them. He thought they all must be on the pill anyway. He never thought of using a condom. He thought AIDS was a gay disease. He found out it is not. He doesn't know if or when he'll actually come down with AIDS, but he does know he's potentially contagious. He's very scared.

C. Bill has AIDS. He's 28. He's been feeling rundown for the past few months and finally went to a doctor to have the purple splotches of skin on his back checked. It is Kaposi's sarcoma. He's been with Mike for almost three years, a relationship they are committed to as being permanent. However, before he met Mike, Bill dated a lot of men. He didn't think about such things as "safe sex" three years ago. He must've gotten AIDS from one of his many intimate partners. He wonders who. Now he's worried about Mike. They haven't been practicing "safe sex" either because they're monogamous. What if Mike has it, too? He truly loves Mike and prays that Mike is all right. Mike's going in for his test results tomorrow. Bill is very worried.

D. Tonya has AIDS. She's 19. She comes from a very poor side of town where living is tough. It seemed everybody was "into" using intravenous drugs. "Shooting up" was easy. Heroin let her escape. Needles were expensive so she shared them with her friends. Now she's very sick. She's in the hospital for some kind of strange pneumonia. This time deep down she doesn't think she'll ever make it home again.

E. Cheryl has AIDS. She's two months old. She got it from her mother who also has it. Cheryl's very weak now. She probably won't last very long.

2. Summarize what has been said and how you could improve your social work skills.

Competencies/Practice Behaviors Exercise 10.6
Everything You Wanted to Know About AIDS, But Were Reluctant to Ask

Focus Competencies or Practice Behaviors:

- EP 2.1.3a Distinguish, appraise, and integrate multiple sources of knowledge, including research-based knowledge and practice wisdom
- EP 2.1.7b Critique and apply knowledge to understand person and environment
- EP 2.1.10a Substantively and affectively prepare for action with individuals, families, groups, organizations, and communities

A. Brief description

You (and the other students) anonymously write down your questions related to AIDS, and the instructor answers them at the next class period.

B. Objectives

You will:

1. Receive answers to questions that you have about AIDS.
2. Better understand the importance of engaging in safe/safer sex practices.

C. Procedure

1. At the end of a class period the instructor distributes note cards to you and the other students, and then asks you (and the other students) to write down questions that you have about AIDS. Students are instructed not to put their names on the cards so that anonymity may be retained.
2. At the next class period the instructor provides answers to the written questions, and also seeks to answer any additional questions that arise.

Chapter 10 Competencies/Practice Behaviors Exercises Assessment:

Name: ______________________________ **Date:** __________
Supervisor's Name: ______________________________

Focus Competencies or Practice Behaviors:

- EP 2.1.1b Practice personal reflection and self-correction to assure continual professional development
- EP 2.1.2a Recognize and manage personal values in a way that allows professional values to guide practice
- EP 2.1.2b Make ethical decisions by applying standards of the National Association of Social Workers Code of Ethics and, as applicable, of the International Federation of Social Workers/International Association of Schools of Social Work Ethics in Social Work, Statement of Principles
- EP 2.1.3a Distinguish, appraise, and integrate multiple sources of knowledge, including research-based knowledge and practice wisdom
- EP 2.1.3b Analyze models of assessment, prevention, intervention, and evaluation
- EP 2.1.6b Use research evidence to inform practice
- EP 2.1.7a Utilize conceptual frameworks to guide the processes of assessment, intervention, and evaluation
- EP 2.1.7b Critique and apply knowledge to understand person and environment
- EP 2.1.10a Substantively and affectively prepare for action with individuals, families, groups, organizations, and communities

Instructions:

A. Evaluate your work or your partner's work in the Focus Competencies/Practice Behaviors by completing the Competencies/Practice Behaviors Assessment form below

B. What other Competencies/Practice Behaviors did you use to complete these Exercises? Be sure to record them in your assessments

1.	I have attained this competency/practice behavior (in the range of 81 to 100%)
2.	I have largely attained this competency/practice behavior (in the range of 61 to 80%)
3.	I have partially attained this competency/practice behavior (in the range of 41 to 60%)
4.	I have made a little progress in attaining this competency/practice behavior (in the range of 21 to 40%)
5.	I have made almost no progress in attaining this competency/practice behavior (in the range of 0 to 20%)

EPAS 2008 Core Competencies & Core Practice Behaviors	Student Self Assessment						Evaluator Feedback
Student and Evaluator Assessment Scale and Comments	**0**	**1**	**2**	**3**	**4**	**5**	**Agree/Disagree/Comments**
EP 2.1.1 Identify as a Professional Social Worker and Conduct Oneself Accordingly:							
a. Advocate for client access to the services of social work							
b. Practice personal reflection and self-correction to assure continual professional development							
c. Attend to professional roles and boundaries							

d. Demonstrate professional demeanor in behavior, appearance, and communication							
e. Engage in career-long learning							
f. Use supervision and consultation							
EP 2.1.2 Apply Social Work Ethical Principles to Guide Professional Practice:							
a. Recognize and manage personal values in a way that allows professional values to guide practice							
b. Make ethical decisions by applying NASW Code of Ethics and, as applicable, of the IFSW/IASSW Ethics in Social Work, Statement of Principles							
c. Tolerate ambiguity in resolving ethical conflicts							
d. Apply strategies of ethical reasoning to arrive at principled decisions							
EP 2.1.3 Apply Critical Thinking to Inform and Communicate Professional Judgments:							
a. Distinguish, appraise, and integrate multiple sources of knowledge, including research-based knowledge and practice wisdom							
b. Analyze models of assessment, prevention, intervention, and evaluation							
c. Demonstrate effective oral and written communication in working with individuals, families, groups, organizations, communities, and colleagues							
EP 2.1.4 Engage Diversity and Difference in Practice:							
a. Recognize the extent to which a culture's structures and values may oppress, marginalize, alienate, or create or enhance privilege and power							
b. Gain sufficient self-awareness to eliminate the influence of personal biases and values in working with diverse groups							
c. Recognize and communicate their understanding of the importance of difference in shaping life experiences							
d. View themselves as learners and engage those with whom they work as informants							
EP 2.1.5 Advance Human Rights and Social and Economic Justice:							
a. Understand forms and mechanisms of oppression and discrimination							
b. Advocate for human rights and social and economic justice							
c. Engage in practices that advance social and economic justice							
EP 2.1.6 Engage in Research-Informed Practice and Practice-Informed Research:							
a. Use practice experience to inform scientific inquiry							
b. Use research evidence to inform practice							
EP 2.1.7 Apply Knowledge of Human Behavior and the Social Environment:							
a. Utilize conceptual frameworks to guide the processes of assessment, intervention, and evaluation							

b. Critique and apply knowledge to understand person and environment							
EP 2.1.8 Engage in Policy Practice to Advance Social and Economic Well-Being and to Deliver Effective Social Work Services:							
a. Analyze, formulate, and advocate for policies that advance social well-being							
b. Collaborate with colleagues and clients for effective policy action							
EP 2.1.9 Respond to Contexts that Shape Practice:							
a. Continuously discover, appraise, and attend to changing locales, populations, scientific and technological developments, and emerging societal trends to provide relevant services							
b. Provide leadership in promoting sustainable changes in service delivery and practice to improve the quality of social services							
EP 2.1.10 Engage, Assess, Intervene, and Evaluate with Individuals, Families, Groups, Organizations and Communities:							
a. Substantively and affectively prepare for action with individuals, families, groups, organizations, and communities							
b. Use empathy and other interpersonal skills							
c. Develop a mutually agreed-on focus of work and desired outcomes							
d. Collect, organize, and interpret client data							
e. Assess client strengths and limitations							
f. Develop mutually agreed-on intervention goals and objectives							
g. Select appropriate intervention strategies							
h. Initiate actions to achieve organizational goals							
i. Implement prevention interventions that enhance client capacities							
j. Help clients resolve problems							
k. Negotiate, mediate, and advocate for clients							
l. Facilitate transitions and endings							
m. Critically analyze, monitor, and evaluate interventions							

Chapter 11
Psychological Aspects of Young and Middle Adulthood

Competencies/Practice Behaviors Exercise 11.1
Assessing Human Behavior

Focus Competencies or Practice Behaviors:

- EP 2.1.1b Practice personal reflection and self-correction to assure continual professional development
- EP 2.1.3a Distinguish, appraise, and integrate multiple sources of knowledge, including research-based knowledge and practice wisdom
- EP 2.1.3b Analyze models of assessment, prevention, intervention, and evaluation
- EP 2.1.3c Demonstrate effective oral and written communication in working with individuals, families, groups, organizations, communities, and colleagues
- EP 2.1.6b Use research evidence to inform practice
- EP 2.1.7a Utilize conceptual frameworks to guide the processes of assessment, intervention, and evaluation
- EP 2.1.7b Critique and apply knowledge to understand person and environment
- EP 2.1.8a Analyze, formulate, and advocate for policies that advance social well-being
- EP 2.1.10a Substantively and affectively prepare for action with individuals, families, groups, organizations, and communities

A. Brief description

You will assess the underlying reasons for unusual behavior you have engaged in using Maslow's theoretical framework, control theory, intuition theory, and the self-talk approach described in chapter 8.

B. Objective

You will:

1. Assess unusual human behavior in terms of Maslow's theoretical framework, game analysis, script analysis, control theory, intuition theory, and the self-talk approach.

C. Procedure

1. Identify something that you did that was highly unusual or bizarre. You need not share what you focus on unless you choose to do so. Your task is to identify the underlying reasons why you did what you did in terms of the following six approaches: (1) Maslow's hierarchy of needs framework, (2) control theory, (3) intuition theory, and (4) self-talk.
2. The instructor briefly describes each of these four approaches. (You should also read the material about these approaches in the text, prior to participating in this exercise.)
3. Silently spend about 15 minutes identifying and writing down the underlying reasons why you did what you did.
4. Volunteers are asked to share what they did and how some or all of these approaches were useful in identifying the underlying reasons for the action.

Competencies/Practice Behaviors Exercise 11.2
Assessing Nonverbal Communication

Focus Competencies or Practice Behaviors:

- EP 2.1.1b Practice personal reflection and self-correction to assure continual professional development
- EP 2.1.3a Distinguish, appraise, and integrate multiple sources of knowledge, including research-based knowledge and practice wisdom
- EP 2.1.3b Analyze models of assessment, prevention, intervention, and evaluation
- EP 2.1.3c Demonstrate effective oral and written communication in working with individuals, families, groups, organizations, communities, and colleagues
- EP 2.1.6b Use research evidence to inform practice
- EP 2.1.7a Utilize conceptual frameworks to guide the processes of assessment, intervention, and evaluation
- EP 2.1.7b Critique and apply knowledge to understand person and environment
- EP 2.1.8a Analyze, formulate, and advocate for policies that advance social well-being
- EP 2.1.10a Substantively and affectively prepare for action with individuals, families, groups, organizations, and communities

A. Brief description

You will assess the nonverbal communication of a relative you dislike and of a relative you like.

B. Objectives

You will:

1. Identify the various ways in which people communicate nonverbally.
2. Identify nonverbal cues you like and dislike.

C. Procedure

1. The instructor begins by describing the purpose of this exercise. Brainstorm about the various ways that people communicate nonverbally, and list these on the chalkboard. A list might include:

Clothing	Gestures and other body movements
Eye movements	Paralanguage
Facial expressions	Use of time
Posture	Eyebrow movements
Physical appearance	Touch
Distance between people communicating	Silence and pauses
Voice tone	Blushing

2. Select a relative you disliked greatly in the past and another you especially liked. Describe on a sheet of paper as specifically as possible what you liked and disliked about the nonverbal communication of each. Avoid listing verbal communication cues, but focus only on nonverbal cues. It is crucial that you do not reveal the names of these relatives in your description, in order to avoid a violation of confidentiality.

3. Volunteers read what they have written. After each description is read, discuss which aspects of the description are nonverbal communication cues and which are not. Also you should seek to arrive at a consensus as to desirable and undesirable nonverbal behaviors for a relative.

Competencies/Practice Behaviors Exercise 11.3
Everything You Always Wanted to Know About Drug Use and Abuse But Were Afraid to Ask

Focus Competencies or Practice Behaviors:

- EP 2.1.1b Practice personal reflection and self-correction to assure continual professional development
- EP 2.1.3a Distinguish, appraise, and integrate multiple sources of knowledge, including research-based knowledge and practice wisdom
- EP 2.1.3b Analyze models of assessment, prevention, intervention, and evaluation
- EP 2.1.3c Demonstrate effective oral and written communication in working with individuals, families, groups, organizations, communities, and colleagues
- EP 2.1.6b Use research evidence to inform practice
- EP 2.1.7a Utilize conceptual frameworks to guide the processes of assessment, intervention, and evaluation
- EP 2.1.7b Critique and apply knowledge to understand person and environment
- EP 2.1.8a Analyze, formulate, and advocate for policies that advance social well-being
- EP 2.1.10a Substantively and affectively prepare for action with individuals, families, groups, organizations, and communities

A. Brief description
You will write questions you have about drug use and abuse, which the instructor will answer at the next class period.

B. Objective
You will:
1. Obtain answers to your personal questions about drug use, abuse, effects, and treatment.

C. Procedure
1. At the end of a class period, anonymously write on a notecard or sheet of paper one or two questions about drugs that you would like answered. Examples of possible questions are:
    a. What are the adverse effects of cocaine use?
    b. How does LSD affect a person?
    c. How do you get a friend or relative to acknowledge a drinking problem?
    d. Is marijuana use more dangerous than use of alcohol?
    e. What kinds of treatment programs are available for those who abuse alcohol or cocaine?
    f. What are the adverse effects of using anabolic steroids?
    g. How can a woman prevent a date rape drug being slipped into her drink?
2. Prior to the next class period the instructor will obtain answers from references or by calling drug counselors.

3. At the next class period the instructor will answer each question, one at a time. You are encouraged to participate in the discussion.

Competencies/Practice Behaviors Exercise 11.4
Communicating While Blindfolded Role-Play

Focus Competencies or Practice Behaviors:

- EP 2.1.1b Practicc personal reflection and self-correction to assure continual professional development
- EP 2.1.3a Distinguish, appraise, and integrate multiple sources of knowledge, including research-based knowledge and practice wisdom
- EP 2.1.3b Analyze models of assessment, prevention, intervention, and evaluation
- EP 2.1.3c Demonstrate effective oral and written communication in working with individuals, families, groups, organizations, communities, and colleagues
- EP 2.1.6b Use research evidence to inform practice
- EP 2.1.7a Utilize conceptual frameworks to guide the processes of assessment, intervention, and evaluation
- EP 2.1.7b Critique and apply knowledge to understand person and environment
- EP 2.1.8a Analyze, formulate, and advocate for policies that advance social well-being
- EP 2.1.10a Substantively and affectively prepare for action with individuals, families, groups, organizations, and communities

A. Brief description

You will discuss a controversial topic in a subgroup while your eyes are closed.

B. Objectives

You will:

1. Better understand how communication is affected when the sense of sight is not used.
2. Be more aware of how nonverbal cues are used in communicating.

C. Procedure

1. The instructor explains that nonverbal communication is heavily dependent on the sense of sight. We watch other people's facial expressions, posture, hand gestures, eyes, and body movements. The instructor describes the objectives of the exercise, and asks the class to form circles of five or six students each. Each subgroup receives a controversial topic to discuss (for example, whether physician-assisted suicide should be legalized in our society). The topic may or may not be the same for each subgroup. All participants are blindfolded and discuss the topic for ten to fifteen minutes. (As an alternative to blindfolding, the instructor may ask the students to keep their eyes closed during the discussion.)
2. At the end of the discussion, the students open their eyes (or remove the blindfolds). One large circle is formed, and the class is asked to discuss the following questions:
   a. How did it feel to communicate with your eyes closed?
   b. How did not being able to see affect the communication?
   c. Did not being able to see interfere with being able to concentrate on what was said?
   d. Did not being able to see result in your missing parts of the verbal messages communicated by others?

e. Do you think you gestured more or less than you usually do?

f. During this exercise did you become more aware of anything that you had not noticed before?

g. Does not being able to see the people you are talking to substantially hamper communication? If yes, in what ways?

Competencies/Practice Behaviors Exercise 11.5
Personal Space Zones

Focus Competencies or Practice Behaviors:

- EP 2.1.1b Practice personal reflection and self-correction to assure continual professional development
- EP 2.1.3a Distinguish, appraise, and integrate multiple sources of knowledge, including research-based knowledge and practice wisdom
- EP 2.1.3b Analyze models of assessment, prevention, intervention, and evaluation
- EP 2.1.3c Demonstrate effective oral and written communication in working with individuals, families, groups, organizations, communities, and colleagues
- EP 2.1.6b Use research evidence to inform practice
- EP 2.1.7a Utilize conceptual frameworks to guide the processes of assessment, intervention, and evaluation
- EP 2.1.7b Critique and apply knowledge to understand person and environment
- EP 2.1.8a Analyze, formulate, and advocate for policies that advance social well-being
- EP 2.1.10a Substantively and affectively prepare for action with individuals, families, groups, organizations, and communities

A. Brief description
Two volunteers talk to each other at varying distances from one another.

B. Objectives
You will:
1. Observe how the distance between communicators affects what people are thinking and feeling.
2. Better understand the concept of personal zones.

C. Procedure
1. The instructor explains the objectives of the exercise, and asks for two volunteers. The volunteers stand at the farthest corners of the room, away from each other. Their task is to slowly—very slowly—walk towards each other. As they are slowly walking towards each other, they engage in small talk about topics of their choosing. They should continue slowly walking and conversing until they touch. When they touch they should slowly start moving apart from each other (while continuing to talk). At the point where they are most comfortable in conversing, they should stop.
2. Other volunteers may be selected to repeat this exercise until interest wanes. The instructor then summarizes the distances at which the various pairs were most comfortable in conversing. The instructor then ends the exercise by discussing the concept of personal zones. The different personal zones are: intimate zone, personal zone, social zone, and public zone.

Chapter 11 Competencies/Practice Behaviors Exercises Assessment:

Name: ______________________________ **Date:** __________
Supervisor's Name: ______________________________

Focus Competencies or Practice Behaviors:

- EP 2.1.1b Practice personal reflection and self-correction to assure continual professional development
- EP 2.1.3a Distinguish, appraise, and integrate multiple sources of knowledge, including research-based knowledge and practice wisdom
- EP 2.1.3b Analyze models of assessment, prevention, intervention, and evaluation
- EP 2.1.3c Demonstrate effective oral and written communication in working with individuals, families, groups, organizations, communities, and colleagues
- EP 2.1.6b Use research evidence to inform practice
- EP 2.1.7a Utilize conceptual frameworks to guide the processes of assessment, intervention, and evaluation
- EP 2.1.7b Critique and apply knowledge to understand person and environment
- EP 2.1.8a Analyze, formulate, and advocate for policies that advance social well-being
- EP 2.1.10a Substantively and affectively prepare for action with individuals, families, groups, organizations, and communities

Instructions:

A. Evaluate your work or your partner's work in the Focus Competencies/Practice Behaviors by completing the Competencies/Practice Behaviors Assessment form below

B. What other Competencies/Practice Behaviors did you use to complete these Exercises? Be sure to record them in your assessments

1.	I have attained this competency/practice behavior (in the range of 81 to 100%)
2.	I have largely attained this competency/practice behavior (in the range of 61 to 80%)
3.	I have partially attained this competency/practice behavior (in the range of 41 to 60%)
4.	I have made a little progress in attaining this competency/practice behavior (in the range of 21 to 40%)
5.	I have made almost no progress in attaining this competency/practice behavior (in the range of 0 to 20%)

EPAS 2008 Core Competencies & Core Practice Behaviors	Student Self Assessment						Evaluator Feedback
Student and Evaluator Assessment Scale and Comments	**0**	**1**	**2**	**3**	**4**	**5**	**Agree/Disagree/Comments**
EP 2.1.1 Identify as a Professional Social Worker and Conduct Oneself Accordingly:							
a. Advocate for client access to the services of social work							
b. Practice personal reflection and self-correction to assure continual professional development							
c. Attend to professional roles and boundaries							
d. Demonstrate professional demeanor in behavior, appearance, and communication							

e. Engage in career-long learning							
f. Use supervision and consultation							
EP 2.1.2 Apply Social Work Ethical Principles to Guide Professional Practice:							
a. Recognize and manage personal values in a way that allows professional values to guide practice							
b. Make ethical decisions by applying NASW Code of Ethics and, as applicable, of the IFSW/IASSW Ethics in Social Work, Statement of Principles							
c. Tolerate ambiguity in resolving ethical conflicts							
d. Apply strategies of ethical reasoning to arrive at principled decisions							
EP 2.1.3 Apply Critical Thinking to Inform and Communicate Professional Judgments:							
a. Distinguish, appraise, and integrate multiple sources of knowledge, including research-based knowledge and practice wisdom							
b. Analyze models of assessment, prevention, intervention, and evaluation							
c. Demonstrate effective oral and written communication in working with individuals, families, groups, organizations, communities, and colleagues							
EP 2.1.4 Engage Diversity and Difference in Practice:							
a. Recognize the extent to which a culture's structures and values may oppress, marginalize, alienate, or create or enhance privilege and power							
b. Gain sufficient self-awareness to eliminate the influence of personal biases and values in working with diverse groups							
c. Recognize and communicate their understanding of the importance of difference in shaping life experiences							
d. View themselves as learners and engage those with whom they work as informants							
EP 2.1.5 Advance Human Rights and Social and Economic Justice:							
a. Understand forms and mechanisms of oppression and discrimination							
b. Advocate for human rights and social and economic justice							
c. Engage in practices that advance social and economic justice							
EP 2.1.6 Engage in Research-Informed Practice and Practice-Informed Research:							
a. Use practice experience to inform scientific inquiry							
b. Use research evidence to inform practice							
EP 2.1.7 Apply Knowledge of Human Behavior and the Social Environment:							
a. Utilize conceptual frameworks to guide the processes of assessment, intervention, and evaluation							
b. Critique and apply knowledge to understand person and environment							

EP 2.1.8 Engage in Policy Practice to Advance Social and Economic Well-Being and to Deliver Effective Social Work Services:							
a. Analyze, formulate, and advocate for policies that advance social well-being							
b. Collaborate with colleagues and clients for effective policy action							
EP 2.1.9 Respond to Contexts that Shape Practice:							
a. Continuously discover, appraise, and attend to changing locales, populations, scientific and technological developments, and emerging societal trends to provide relevant services							
b. Provide leadership in promoting sustainable changes in service delivery and practice to improve the quality of social services							
EP 2.1.10 Engage, Assess, Intervene, and Evaluate with Individuals, Families, Groups, Organizations and Communities:							
a. Substantively and affectively prepare for action with individuals, families, groups, organizations, and communities							
b. Use empathy and other interpersonal skills							
c. Develop a mutually agreed-on focus of work and desired outcomes							
d. Collect, organize, and interpret client data							
e. Assess client strengths and limitations							
f. Develop mutually agreed-on intervention goals and objectives							
g. Select appropriate intervention strategies							
h. Initiate actions to achieve organizational goals							
i. Implement prevention interventions that enhance client capacities							
j. Help clients resolve problems							
k. Negotiate, mediate, and advocate for clients							
l. Facilitate transitions and endings							
m. Critically analyze, monitor, and evaluate interventions							

Chapter 12
Sociological Aspects of Young and Middle Adulthood

Competencies/Practice Behaviors Exercise 12.1
Assessing Intimate Relationships

Focus Competencies or Practice Behaviors:

- EP 2.1.1b Practice personal reflection and self-correction to assure continual professional development
- EP 2.1.3b Analyze models of assessment, prevention, intervention, and evaluation
- EP 2.1.6b Use research evidence to inform practice
- EP 2.1.7b Critique and apply knowledge to understand person and environment

A. Brief description

You will evaluate some aspects of an intimate relationship you have had by answering various questions confidentially. Discussion then focuses on critical issues involved in the assessment of relationships.

B. Objectives

You will:

1. Identify some of the basic issues involved in intimate relationships.
2. Examine the difficulty of relationship assessment.
3. Relate your own life experience to the experience of others.

C. Procedure

1. Picture a time in your life (which may be the present) when you were involved in an intimate relationship. Complete the following statements and answer the questions on the basis of that relationship. The questions resemble those often used to assess the functioning of a couple that has requested counseling. It is helpful to discuss and complete each section independently.

SECTION A: EXPLORATION

1. If I were to describe our relationship in one word, it would be ___.
2. My partner and I are alike in the way that we ___.
3. My partner and I are different in that we ___.
4. If our relationship were a television movie, the title would be ___.
5. The needs my partner fulfills for me are ___.
6. The needs that my partner does not fulfill for me are ___.
7. The things my partner does that please me include ___.
8. The things my partner does that annoy me include ___.
9. I am proud of my partner when ___.
10. My partner is proud of me when ___.
11. I feel that my partner's and my ability to talk and communicate with each other is ___.
12. The things I would like to talk to my partner about, but don't, include ___.

13. My major concern in our relationship is ___.
14. I think my partner's major concern in our relationship is ___.
15. When my partner and I have conflicts, we ___.
16. I wish my partner would tell me ___.
17. The thing I think my partner would like to know about me is ___.
18. I have the most fun with my partner when ___.
19. I have the least fun with my partner when ___.
20. I would like our relationship to ___.

SECTION B: SPECIFYING STRENGTHS AND WEAKNESSES

My major strengths are:

1.

2.

3.

4.

5.

My partner's major strengths are:

1.

2.

3.

4.

5.

My major weaknesses are:

1.

2.

3.

4.

5.

My partner's major weaknesses are:

1.

2.

3.

4.

5.

SECTION C: CHANGES AND GOALS

The changes I would like to see in our relationship (in order of priority) are:

1.

2.

3.

The changes I think my partner would like to see (in order of what I think my partner's priorities would be) are:

1.

2.

3.

Immediate goals I would like to strive for in our relationship are:

1.

2.

Long-term goals I would like to strive for in our relationship are:

1.

2.

2. After each section, answer the following or similar questions:
   a. What are your reactions to the exercise?
   b. How did you feel while answering the questions?
   c. How difficult did you think the exercise was?
   d. What were the reasons for any difficulties you encountered?
   e. How might a couple seeking counseling because of relationship problems feel when asked such questions?
   f. What did you learn from doing this exercise?

Competencies/Practice Behaviors Exercise 12.2
Romantic Love Versus Rational Love

Focus Competencies or Practice Behaviors:

- EP 2.1.1b Practice personal reflection and self-correction to assure continual professional development
- EP 2.1.3b Analyze models of assessment, prevention, intervention, and evaluation
- EP 2.1.6b Use research evidence to inform practice
- EP 2.1.7a Utilize conceptual frameworks to guide the processes of assessment, intervention, and evaluation
- EP 2.1.7b Critique and apply knowledge to understand person and environment

A. Brief description

You will analyze a current or past love relationship to determine whether the attraction was primarily a romantic love relationship or a rational love relationship.

B. Objectives

You will:

1. Learn how to analyze the positives and negatives in love relationships.
2. Assess the nature of attraction in love relationships.

C. Procedure

1. Write down on a sheet of paper the following information about someone with whom you are currently "in love." If you are not currently in a love relationship, then write about someone you were "in love" with in the past. The information you write will be confidential. You will not be asked to share this information with anyone.

The items or characteristics that I find (or found) attractive about this person are:	The items or characteristics that I find (or found) irritating about this person are:
1.	1.
2.	2.
3.	3.
4.	4.
5.	5.
6.	6.

2. The instructor explains the characteristics of romantic relationships and rational love relationships, and describes the pitfalls of romantic love. (This material is presented in the text.)
3. Examine what you wrote, and silently assess whether your relationship is (was) primarily one of romantic love or rational love. If you listed all positives about your partner, you probably are idealizing your partner, and therefore the relationship is apt to be a romantic love relationship. If you listed both positives and irritants, you are apt to be in a rational love relationship. If you listed all irritants, then your love relationship may have ended, or be near ending.
4. Discuss the merits and shortcomings of analyzing love relationships in terms of the conceptualization of romantic love versus rational love.

Competencies/Practice Behaviors Exercise 12.3
Attitudes Toward Marriage and Divorce

Focus Competencies or Practice Behaviors:

- EP 2.1.1b Practice personal reflection and self-correction to assure continual professional development
- EP 2.1.2a Recognize and manage personal values in a way that allows professional values to guide practice
- EP 2.1.6b Use research evidence to inform practice
- EP 2.1.7b Critique and apply knowledge to understand person and environment

A. Brief description

You will anonymously fill out an attitudinal questionnaire, and the responses will then be discussed.

B. Objectives

You will:

1. Become more aware of your attitudes and values toward marriage and divorce.
2. Become more aware of your attitudes toward physical abuse.

C. Procedure

1. You are asked questions related to your attitudes toward marriage, spouse abuse, and divorce. Paper or 5" by 7" notecards are distributed on which to record the answers. Number from 1 through 15 on the response sheet. <u>DO NOT</u> write your name on the sheet.
2. The instructor reads the following questions, giving you time to record your responses.

a. If a man is drunk and yelling obscenities at his wife, do you think the woman has a right to slap his face in order to get him to stop yelling obscenities?
____ Yes ____ No

b. If a woman discovers that her husband is having an affair with someone else, do you think she has a right to show her indignation by slapping his face?
____ Yes ____ No

c. If you were in an empty-shell marriage, would you choose to get a divorce over maintaining the marriage?
____ Yes ____ No

d. In a marriage where there is considerable tension and discord, are the children generally better off psychologically if a divorce is obtained?
____ Yes ____ No

e. If you were married to someone and discovered that your spouse had had several affairs while married, would you seriously consider getting a divorce?
____ Yes ____ No

f. If you were married to someone who became permanently paralyzed from the neck down in an automobile accident, would you seriously consider getting a divorce?
____ Yes ____ No

g. If you were married to someone who became chronically depressed and suicidal, would you seriously consider getting a divorce?
____ Yes ____ No

h. If you were married to someone who periodically physically abused you or other family members, would you seriously consider getting a divorce?
____ Yes ____ No

i. If you were married to someone and then discovered your spouse was primarily homosexual in sexual orientation, would you seriously consider getting a divorce?
____ Yes ____ No

j. If you were married to someone who developed such a severe drinking problem that he or she was unable to hold a job, would you seriously consider getting a divorce?

____ Yes ____ No

k. If you were married to someone who tested HIV positive and you are HIV negative, would you seriously consider getting a divorce?

____ Yes ____ No

l. If a man discovers that his wife is having an affair with someone else, do you think the man has a right to show his indignation by slapping his wife's face?

____ Yes ____ No

m. If a woman is drunk and is yelling obscenities at her husband, do you think the husband has a right to slap the woman's face in order to get her to stop yelling obscenities?

____ Yes ____ No

n. Have you ever been slapped or hit by someone you were romantically involved with?

____ Yes ____ No

o. Have you ever slapped or hit someone you were romantically involved with?

____ Yes ____ No

3. The instructor collects the responses. The letters a through o are listed on the board. Volunteers record the responses of the students.
4. The instructor reads each question aloud and the responses are noted and discussed.

Competencies/Practice Behaviors Exercise 12.4
Poverty Functionalism Versus Conflict Theory

Focus Competencies or Practice Behaviors:

- EP 2.1.1b Practice personal reflection and self-correction to assure continual professional development
- EP 2.1.6b Use research evidence to inform practice
- EP 2.1.7a Utilize conceptual frameworks to guide the processes of assessment, intervention, and evaluation
- EP 2.1.7b Critique and apply knowledge to understand person and environment
- EP 2.1.8a Analyze, formulate, and advocate for policies that advance social well-being

A. Brief description

You will discuss questions about poverty that are generated by functionalism and conflict theory.

B. Objectives

You will:

1. Describe functionalism and conflict theory.
2. Analyze poverty in terms of functionalism and conflict theory.

C. Procedure

1. The instructor describes the vast differences in income and wealth that exist in our society. He or she defines functionalism and conflict theory, summarizes the proposals of each for reducing poverty, and describes the controversial notion that poverty may be functional for the rich.
2. The instructor writes the following questions on the board, or you may read the questions in this manual:
   a. Do you believe poverty is functional for our society?
   b. Since poverty could virtually be eliminated in our society by a redistribution of wealth and income from the rich to the poor, do you believe the existing power structure really wants to eliminate poverty?
   c. Do you believe the poor are largely to blame for being poor, or do you believe poverty is largely due to societal factors that are beyond the control of the poor?
   d. Which do you believe has better ideas on how to reduce poverty in our society—functionalism or conflict theory?
3. Form groups of five or six. You have 10 to 15 minutes to arrive at answers to these questions. Then share your opinions. After each subgroup presents its positions, discuss the merits and shortcomings of these positions.

Competencies/Practice Behaviors Exercise 12.5
Liberalism Versus Conservatism Role-Play

Focus Competencies or Practice Behaviors:

- EP 2.1.3a Distinguish, appraise, and integrate multiple sources of knowledge, including research-based knowledge and practice wisdom
- EP 2.1.3b Analyze models of assessment, prevention, intervention, and evaluation
- EP 2.1.6b Use research evidence to inform practice
- EP 2.1.7a Utilize conceptual frameworks to guide the processes of assessment, intervention, and evaluation
- EP 2.1.7b Critique and apply knowledge to understand person and environment
- EP 2.1.8a Analyze, formulate, and advocate for policies that advance social well-being
- EP 2.1.8b Collaborate with colleagues and clients for effective policy action
- EP 2.1.9a Continuously discover, appraise, and attend to changing locales, populations, scientific and technological developments, and emerging societal trends to provide relevant services
- EP 2.1.9b Provide leadership in promoting sustainable changes in service delivery and practice to improve the quality of social services

A. Brief description

You will discuss the two prominent political philosophies in the United States: liberalism and conservatism. You will also discuss the applications of these two approaches to resolving social problems. Finally, you will discuss the developmental perspective which is an emerging perspective that has appeal to both liberals and conservatives.

B. Objectives
You will:
1. Understand and describe liberalism, conservatism, and the developmental perspective.
2. Present arguments as to which approach has the most potential for resolving contemporary social problems.

C. Procedure
1. Read the descriptive material on liberalism, conservatism, and the developmental perspective in the text. The instructor may choose to begin the exercise by summarizing the basic postulates of these philosophies. (Have your textbook available in class to use for reference.)
2. Form subgroups of five or six persons. The instructor distributes a notecard with a social problem written on it to each subgroup. Each subgroup is given a different social problem. You have 20 minutes to arrive at a consensus as to how liberals, conservatives, and those who adhere to the developmental perspective would combat the social problem listed on your notecard. Each group should also arrive at a consensus on whether liberals, conservatives, or those who adhere to the developmental perspective have the better approach for resolving the specified social problem.
3. One or two representatives from each group present to the class (a) the liberal, conservative, and developmental approaches to resolving the specified social problem, and (b) the group's views as to which of these three perspectives have the better approach to resolving the social problem.

Competencies/Practice Behaviors Exercise 12.6
Needed Services for Blended Families

Focus Competencies or Practice Behaviors:

- EP 2.1.1a Advocate for client access to the services of social work
- EP 2.1.3a Distinguish, appraise, and integrate multiple sources of knowledge, including research-based knowledge and practice wisdom
- EP 2.1.6b Use research evidence to inform practice
- EP 2.1.7b Critique and apply knowledge to understand person and environment
- EP 2.1.8a Analyze, formulate, and advocate for policies that advance social well-being
- EP 2.1.8b Collaborate with colleagues and clients for effective policy action
- EP 2.1.9a Continuously discover, appraise, and attend to changing locales, populations, scientific and technological developments, and emerging societal trends to provide relevant services

A. Brief description
You will identify problems encountered by blended families and then recommend needed services to assist blended families in handling these problems.

B. Objectives
You will:
1. Become more knowledgeable about the needs of blended families.
2. Become more aware of services to meet these needs.

C. Procedure

1. Blended families are becoming a typical family form in our society, and there is only limited information available on the problems encountered by these families and on the social services needed by these families. The instructor will either have you read the material on blended families in the text or will summarize this material in a brief lecture.
2. Form groups of about five persons. First identify what you view as being the four or five most difficult or serious problems encountered by blended families. After you have completed this task, identify the social services that would help blended families handle these problems.

Competencies/Practice Behaviors Exercise 12.7
An Ecomap of My Family

Focus Competencies or Practice Behaviors:

- EP 2.1.1b Practice personal reflection and self-correction to assure continual professional development
- EP 2.1.7a Utilize conceptual frameworks to guide the processes of assessment, intervention, and evaluation

A. Brief description

You will draw an ecomap of your family. Volunteers will share their ecomap with the class.

B. Objectives

You will:

1. Practice this family system assessment technique.
2. Gain insight into the dynamics of your family.

C. Procedure

1. The instructor distributes large sheets of paper and magic markers. Using the symbols and instructions in the text, draw an ecomap of your family.
2. Volunteers describe their ecomaps.

Competencies/Practice Behaviors Exercise 12.8
A Genogram of My Family

Focus Competencies or Practice Behaviors:

- EP 2.1.1b Practice personal reflection and self-correction to assure continual professional development
- EP 2.1.7a Utilize conceptual frameworks to guide the processes of assessment, intervention, and evaluation

A. Brief description

A genogram is essentially a family tree. You will draw a genogram of your family. Volunteers will share their genograms with the class. (The instructions for this exercise are similar to Exercise 7. There are a number of similarities between eco-maps and genograms.)

B. Objectives

You will:

1. Comprehend the family system assessment value of a genogram.
2. Gain insight into dynamics of your family and its history.

C. Procedure

1. The instructor distributes large sheets of paper and magic markers to you and the other students. Using the symbols and instructions in the text, draw a genogram of your family.
2. Volunteers share and describe their genograms.

Competencies/Practice Behaviors Exercise 12.9
Analyzing the Stages in a Love Relationship

Focus Competencies or Practice Behaviors:

- EP 2.1.1b Practice personal reflection and self-correction to assure continual professional development
- EP 2.1.7a Utilize conceptual frameworks to guide the processes of assessment, intervention, and evaluation
- EP 2.1.7b Critique and apply knowledge to understand person and environment

A. Brief description

Analyze a love relationship in terms of Cameron-Bandler's framework, which is described in the text, and reflect on suggestions for improving love relationships.

B. Objectives

You will:

1. Analyze love relationships.
2. Become aware of guidelines or suggestions for improving love relationships.

C. Procedure

1. The instructor describes Cameron-Bandler's framework of the stages in a love relationship (described in the text). Reflect on a love relationship you currently have or had in the past. Silently identify to yourself what stage you are now at in the relationship.
2. The instructor summarizes suggestions (described in the text) for improving love relationships. Silently reflect on whether any of these suggestions are useful for improving your current relationship or might have been useful in improving a relationship you had in the past.
3. Form small groups of about five and share only what you feel comfortable in sharing related to your responses to the questions that were asked in the above steps.
4. After this discussion, the instructor asks if any subgroup wants to share with the class what it discussed. Are there any comments on the merits and shortcomings of this exercise?

Competencies/Practice Behaviors Exercise 12.10
Resolving Interpersonal Conflicts

Focus Competencies or Practice Behaviors:

- EP 2.1.1b Practice personal reflection and self-correction to assure continual professional development
- EP 2.1.7a Utilize conceptual frameworks to guide the processes of assessment, intervention, and evaluation
- EP 2.1.7b Critique and apply knowledge to understand person and environment
- EP 2.1.10a Substantively and affectively prepare for action with individuals, families, groups, organizations, and communities

A. Brief description

Examine a recent interpersonal conflict, and then reflect on whether other conflict resolution strategies would be more effective in resolving the conflict.

B. Objectives

You will:

1. Become aware of a variety of conflict resolution strategies.
2. Become more skillful in resolving future interpersonal conflicts.

C. Procedure

1. Students are instructed to write down on a sheet of paper a summary of a recent interpersonal conflict that they had—perhaps involving a friend, a relative, another student, or a faculty member. The summary should include who the conflict was with, what was at issue, and how it was resolved. (If the issue has not been resolved, the summary should contain a description of the current status of the conflict.)
2. The instructor describes the following conflict resolution strategies and lists them on the chalkboard: the win-lose approach, the problem-solving approach, role reversal, empathy, inquiry, assertiveness, I-messages, disarming, stroking, and mediation.
3. The class forms into subgroups of three students each. The subgroups share with each other the nature of the interpersonal conflicts they summarized in step 1. (Students have a right not to reveal what they wrote.) For each conflict that is shared in the subgroup, the members discuss whether <u>needs</u> or <u>solutions</u> of the people involved in the conflict were primarily at issue. The subgroups also discuss whether any of the following strategies were used (or would have been helpful to use) in resolving the various conflicts: the problem-solving approach, role reversal, empathy, inquiry, assertiveness, I-messages, disarming, stroking, and/or mediation.
4. The class re-forms, and students are given an opportunity to ask questions about conflict resolution. Some students may want to share a complicated unresolved conflict situation they are now experiencing in order to obtain feedback on how it may be effectively resolved.

Competencies/Practice Behaviors Exercise 12.11
Analyzing a Human Services Organization

Focus Competencies or Practice Behaviors:

- EP 2.1.7a Utilize conceptual frameworks to guide the processes of assessment, intervention, and evaluation
- EP 2.1.10a Substantively and affectively prepare for action with individuals, families, groups, organizations, and communities

A. Brief description
You visit a human services organization and gather information to write a report, according to formatted questions, about the organization.

B. Objectives
You will:
1. Learn an approach to analyzing a human services organization.
2. Acquire valuable information about the agency you visit.

C. Procedure
1. Each student visits (perhaps in groups of two or three) a human services agency and writes a report covering the following information. (Some agencies may not have information or data on one or more questions. If the information in unavailable, the students should indicate this in their reports.)

a. What is the agency's mission statement?
b. What are its clients' major problems?
c. What services does the agency provide?
d. How are client needs determined?
e. What percentage of clients are people of color, women, gays or lesbians, elderly, or members of other at-risk populations?
f. What was the total cost of services for the past year?
g. How much money is spent on each program?
h. What are the agency's funding sources?
i. How much and what percentage of funds are received from each source?
j. What types of clients does the agency refuse?
k. What other agencies provide the same services in the community?
l. What is the organizational structure of the agency? For example, is there a formal chain of command?
m. Is there an informal organization (that is, people who exert a greater amount of influence on decision making than would be expected for their formal position in the bureaucracy)?
n. How much decision-making input do the direct service providers have on major policy decisions?
o. Does the agency have a board that oversees its operations? If yes, what are the backgrounds of the board members?
p. Do employees at every level feel valued?
q. What is the morale among employees?

r. What are the major unmet needs of the agency?
s. Does the agency have a handbook of personnel policies and procedures?
t. What is the public image of the agency in the community?
u. In recent years what has been the rate of turnover among staff at the agency? What were the major reasons for leaving?
v. Does the agency have a process for evaluating the outcomes of its services? If yes, what is the process, and what are the outcome results?
w. What is the student's overall impression of the agency? For example, if the student needed services that this agency provides, would she or he want to apply at this agency? Why, or why not?

2. The reports are handed in, on a specified date, to the instructor.

Competencies/Practice Behaviors Exercise 12.12
Theory X Versus Theory Y

Focus Competencies or Practice Behaviors:

- EP 2.1.1b Practice personal reflection and self-correction to assure continual professional development
- EP 2.1.6b Use research evidence to inform practice
- EP 2.1.7a Utilize conceptual frameworks to guide the processes of assessment, intervention, and evaluation
- EP 2.1.7b Critique and apply knowledge to understand person and environment

A. Brief description
You will analyze the benefits and shortcomings of two contrasting management styles—Theory X versus Theory Y.

B. Objectives
You will:
1. Gain an understanding of two contrasting management styles.
2. Be able to analyze management styles in terms of these two contrasting theories.

C. Procedure
1. The instructor explains the objectives of this exercise and describes both Theory X and Theory Y styles of management, providing examples of personal employment under a manager who used one or the other style.
2. You (and the other students in the class) are encouraged to describe examples of employment experiences you have had under these styles and to share your feelings about these contrasting styles.
3. You (and the other students) are encouraged to discuss the merits and shortcomings of these contrasting styles.

Chapter 12 Competencies/Practice Behaviors Exercises Assessment:

Name: ______________________________ **Date:** ________
Supervisor's Name: ____________________

Focus Competencies or Practice Behaviors:

- EP 2.1.1a Advocate for client access to the services of social work
- EP 2.1.1b Practice personal reflection and self-correction to assure continual professional development
- EP 2.1.2a Recognize and manage personal values in a way that allows professional values to guide practice
- EP 2.1.3a Distinguish, appraise, and integrate multiple sources of knowledge, including research-based knowledge and practice wisdom
- EP 2.1.3b Analyze models of assessment, prevention, intervention, and evaluation
- EP 2.1.6b Use research evidence to inform practice
- EP 2.1.7a Utilize conceptual frameworks to guide the processes of assessment, intervention, and evaluation
- EP 2.1.7b Critique and apply knowledge to understand person and environment
- EP 2.1.8a Analyze, formulate, and advocate for policies that advance social well-being
- EP 2.1.8b Collaborate with colleagues and clients for effective policy action
- EP 2.1.9a Continuously discover, appraise, and attend to changing locales, populations, scientific and technological developments, and emerging societal trends to provide relevant services
- EP 2.1.9b Provide leadership in promoting sustainable changes in service delivery and practice to improve the quality of social services
- EP 2.1.10a Substantively and affectively prepare for action with individuals, families, groups, organizations, and communities

Instructions:

A. Evaluate your work or your partner's work in the Focus Competencies/Practice Behaviors by completing the Competencies/Practice Behaviors Assessment form below

B. What other Competencies/Practice Behaviors did you use to complete these Exercises? Be sure to record them in your assessments

1.	I have attained this competency/practice behavior (in the range of 81 to 100%)
2.	I have largely attained this competency/practice behavior (in the range of 61 to 80%)
3.	I have partially attained this competency/practice behavior (in the range of 41 to 60%)
4.	I have made a little progress in attaining this competency/practice behavior (in the range of 21 to 40%)
5.	I have made almost no progress in attaining this competency/practice behavior (in the range of 0 to 20%)

EPAS 2008 Core Competencies & Core Practice Behaviors	Student Self Assessment						Evaluator Feedback
Student and Evaluator Assessment Scale and Comments	**0**	**1**	**2**	**3**	**4**	**5**	**Agree/Disagree/Comments**
EP 2.1.1 Identify as a Professional Social Worker and Conduct Oneself Accordingly:							
a. Advocate for client access to the services of social work							

b.	Practice personal reflection and self-correction to assure continual professional development							
c.	Attend to professional roles and boundaries							
d.	Demonstrate professional demeanor in behavior, appearance, and communication							
e.	Engage in career-long learning							
f.	Use supervision and consultation							
EP 2.1.2 Apply Social Work Ethical Principles to Guide Professional Practice:								
a.	Recognize and manage personal values in a way that allows professional values to guide practice							
b.	Make ethical decisions by applying NASW Code of Ethics and, as applicable, of the IFSW/IASSW Ethics in Social Work, Statement of Principles							
c.	Tolerate ambiguity in resolving ethical conflicts							
d.	Apply strategies of ethical reasoning to arrive at principled decisions							
EP 2.1.3 Apply Critical Thinking to Inform and Communicate Professional Judgments:								
a.	Distinguish, appraise, and integrate multiple sources of knowledge, including research-based knowledge and practice wisdom							
b.	Analyze models of assessment, prevention, intervention, and evaluation							
c.	Demonstrate effective oral and written communication in working with individuals, families, groups, organizations, communities, and colleagues							
EP 2.1.4 Engage Diversity and Difference in Practice:								
a.	Recognize the extent to which a culture's structures and values may oppress, marginalize, alienate, or create or enhance privilege and power							
b.	Gain sufficient self-awareness to eliminate the influence of personal biases and values in working with diverse groups							
c.	Recognize and communicate their understanding of the importance of difference in shaping life experiences							
d.	View themselves as learners and engage those with whom they work as informants							
EP 2.1.5 Advance Human Rights and Social and Economic Justice:								
a.	Understand forms and mechanisms of oppression and discrimination							
b.	Advocate for human rights and social and economic justice							
c.	Engage in practices that advance social and economic justice							
EP 2.1.6 Engage in Research-Informed Practice and Practice-Informed Research:								
a.	Use practice experience to inform scientific inquiry							
b.	Use research evidence to inform practice							

EP 2.1.7 Apply Knowledge of Human Behavior and the Social Environment:							
a. Utilize conceptual frameworks to guide the processes of assessment, intervention, and evaluation							
b. Critique and apply knowledge to understand person and environment							
EP 2.1.8 Engage in Policy Practice to Advance Social and Economic Well-Being and to Deliver Effective Social Work Services:							
a. Analyze, formulate, and advocate for policies that advance social well-being							
b. Collaborate with colleagues and clients for effective policy action							
EP 2.1.9 Respond to Contexts that Shape Practice:							
a. Continuously discover, appraise, and attend to changing locales, populations, scientific and technological developments, and emerging societal trends to provide relevant services							
b. Provide leadership in promoting sustainable changes in service delivery and practice to improve the quality of social services							
EP 2.1.10 Engage, Assess, Intervene, and Evaluate with Individuals, Families, Groups, Organizations and Communities:							
a. Substantively and affectively prepare for action with individuals, families, groups, organizations, and communities							
b. Use empathy and other interpersonal skills							
c. Develop a mutually agreed-on focus of work and desired outcomes							
d. Collect, organize, and interpret client data							
e. Assess client strengths and limitations							
f. Develop mutually agreed-on intervention goals and objectives							
g. Select appropriate intervention strategies							
h. Initiate actions to achieve organizational goals							
i. Implement prevention interventions that enhance client capacities							
j. Help clients resolve problems							
k. Negotiate, mediate, and advocate for clients							
l. Facilitate transitions and endings							
m. Critically analyze, monitor, and evaluate interventions							

Chapter 13
Sexual Orientation

Competencies/Practice Behaviors Exercise 13.1
If I Woke Up Gay Tomorrow Morning . . .

Focus Competencies or Practice Behaviors:

- EP 2.1.4a Recognize the extent to which a culture's structures and values may oppress, marginalize, alienate, or create or enhance privilege and power
- EP 2.1.4b Gain sufficient self-awareness to eliminate the influence of personal biases and values in working with diverse groups
- EP 2.1.4c Recognize and communicate their understanding of the importance of difference in shaping life experiences
- EP 2.1.5a Understand forms and mechanisms of oppression and discrimination

A. Brief description
The class will divide into small groups. You will discuss how you would feel if you woke up lesbian or gay tomorrow morning. Implications are discussed.

B. Objectives
You will:
1. Identify some of the issues confronting lesbian and gay people today.
2. Examine your own feelings and ideas about homosexuality.
3. Formulate and evaluate some of the viable alternatives available to lesbian and gay people today.

C. Procedure
1. Form groups of four to six people.
2. Discuss the following questions. It's important that all group members participate in the discussion and share answers. Choose one person to summarize responses to share with the class.
   a. "How would your life be different if you woke up tomorrow morning and discovered you were lesbian or gay?"
   b. "How would this affect your relationships with friends, family, and colleagues?"
   c. "To whom would you come out and how?"
   d. "How would this affect your social and work life?"
3. You will have 10 to 15 minutes to discuss the question.
4. Ask a volunteer to summarize your group's discussion and share this summary with the larger group.
5. Finally, formulate a summary statement regarding the conclusions of the entire class.

Competencies/Practice Behaviors Exercise 13.2
Am I Homosexual?

Focus Competencies or Practice Behaviors:

- EP 2.1.1b Practice personal reflection and self-correction to assure continual professional development
- EP 2.1.2a Recognize and manage personal values in a way that allows professional values to guide practice
- EP 2.1.4a Recognize the extent to which a culture's structures and values may oppress, marginalize, alienate, or create or enhance privilege and power
- EP 2.1.4b Gain sufficient self-awareness to eliminate the influence of personal biases and values in working with diverse groups
- EP 2.1.4c Recognize and communicate their understanding of the importance of difference in shaping life experiences

A. Brief description

The instructor will read a series of vignettes. You are then asked whether you think the vignettes are about homosexuals. Discussion follows.

B. Objectives

You will:

1. Question some of your basic assumptions about being lesbian or gay.
2. Evaluate your stereotypes about being lesbian or gay.
3. Examine the difficulty involved in defining homosexuality.

C. Procedure

1. The following vignettes are read to the class:

a. I am a 30-year-old female librarian. I love my work and consider myself a dedicated professional. I'm not really very attractive and am about twenty-five pounds overweight. I'm shy and don't have many friends. I'm pretty lonely most of the time. I dated a man in college, but he dropped me to go out with somebody else. I really have never had any other boyfriends. A woman I work with has approached me about having a sexual relationship with her. I'm kind of afraid, but I'm really considering getting involved with her. It sure gets lonely on Saturday nights. Am I a lesbian?

b. I am a 30-year-old man. I've been in prison for six years now for murder. I'm serving a life sentence and really don't know if I'll ever get out on parole. I'm married and still love my wife. We had a good sexual relationship before I came to jail. Here I've had hundreds of sexual relationships with men. I have to admit I do enjoy them and get sexual satisfaction out of them. Am I gay?

c. I am a 30-year-old married man. My wife takes very good care of me sexually on a regular basis. I enjoy our sexual relationship very much. Whenever I have sex with her I like to fantasize about having sex with a man. I also like to watch male wrestlers on television. It's sexually exciting to me. They really turn me on. Am I gay?

2. After you have discussed each vignette, join a general discussion concerning the difficulty of defining homosexuality and the many gradations of homosexual and heterosexual behavior that are possible.

Competencies/Practice Behaviors Exercise 13.3
My Friend is Coming to Visit Role-Play

Focus Competencies or Practice Behaviors:

- EP 2.1.4a Recognize the extent to which a culture's structures and values may oppress, marginalize, alienate, or create or enhance privilege and power
- EP 2.1.4b Gain sufficient self-awareness to eliminate the influence of personal biases and values in working with diverse groups
- EP 2.1.4c Recognize and communicate their understanding of the importance of difference in shaping life experiences
- EP 2.1.5a Understand forms and mechanisms of oppression and discrimination
- EP 2.1.5b Advocate for human rights and social and economic justice

A. Brief description

You will be asked to participate in a role-play: a college junior announces to his or her roommates that a lover of the same gender is coming to visit. Class discussion follows observation of the role-play.

B. Objectives

You will:

1. Recognize some of the difficulties in "coming out" to those close to you.
2. Examine some of the dynamics involved in homophobia.
3. Confront and assess your own values concerning gay and lesbian people.

C. Procedure

1. Six volunteers are needed to dramatize a "coming out" situation.
2. Focus on the following six roles:

The Person Coming Out: You are a college student living in the same house with five other students. Although you all have been housemates for a year, none of the others knows that you are gay. You have invited your lover, who is of the same gender, to stay the weekend with you. You need to tell your housemates about it.

Housemate 1: You don't know much about homosexuality, although you've heard many dirty jokes about it. You really don't know how you feel about it because you've never knowingly met a lesbian or gay person.

Housemate 2: You are very religious and belong to a conservative denomination. You believe that homosexuality is a sin.

Housemate 3: You are a psychology major who sees homosexuality as a *paraphilia* ("recurring, intense, unconventional sexual fantasies, urges, or behavior that is obsessive and compulsive") or illness (Hyde & Delamater, 2008, p. G-6). You think that lesbian and gay people need counseling so that they can become "normal."

Housemate 4: You see sexual orientation as something an individual has the right to choose. You have several gay friends of both sexes. Their sexual orientation is irrelevant to you. You see homosexuality as simply one aspect of an individual's personality.

Housemate 5: You have never really thought much about homosexuality. However, in general you feel that it restricts people's relationships and their life-style. You feel sorry for people who are "that way."

3. Role-players should put themselves into their respective parts and play each individual's attitudes as closely to the part as possible. They may add any other facts as they wish. It's important to remain in the respective roles until the role-play is over. The role-play should last for approximately 15 minutes.
4. After terminating the role-play, both role-players and class observers can discuss the following questions:
   a. What were the reactions of role-players to their respective roles?
   b. How did it feel and how did you think it might feel to be the person coming out? What were the observers' reactions to each respective role?
   c. What are your perceptions of the individual rights, group rights, and social pressure involved?
   d. What do you think would be the "right" thing for each of the role-players to do in such a situation?

Competencies/Practice Behaviors Exercise 13.4
What it Means to be Lesbian or Gay

Focus Competencies or Practice Behaviors:

- EP 2.1.1b Practice personal reflection and self-correction to assure continual professional development
- EP 2.1.2a Recognize and manage personal values in a way that allows professional values to guide practice
- EP 2.1.4a Recognize the extent to which a culture's structures and values may oppress, marginalize, alienate, or create or enhance privilege and power
- EP 2.1.4b Gain sufficient self-awareness to eliminate the influence of personal biases and values in working with diverse groups
- EP 2.1.4c Recognize and communicate their understanding of the importance of difference in shaping life experiences
- EP 2.1.5a Understand forms and mechanisms of oppression and discrimination

A. Brief description
You will be asked to identify some aspect of your life that is very important to you and examine how you would feel if you had to give it up.

B. Objectives
You will:
1. Begin to recognize the difficulty gay and lesbian people have living in a heterosexual world.
2. Examine what being gay or lesbian means to an individual.

C. Procedure

1. Think carefully about what aspect of your life is the most meaningful to you. It could be an activity you heartily enjoy, a goal you are sincerely committed to achieve, a very special person, or some personality characteristic about which you are very proud. Take a piece of scratch paper and jot the life aspect down.
2. Now imagine that you have to live without that part of yourself or your life forever. What would it be like? How would you feel? What would you do without it?
3. You have two or three minutes to think about what giving up such a significant part of your life would be like. Then begin a class discussion focusing on the following questions and issues:
   a. What part of your life did you choose to give up?
   b. How meaningful is that life aspect to you?
   c. How did it feel to even think about giving it up?
   d. Did you think about the potential painfulness of living without this part of your life?
   e. To what extent do you think giving up the life aspect that is particularly important to you would be like giving up being gay or lesbian?
4. Discuss how difficult it would be to change something that is a part of your core self. To what extent could you change your orientation, for any reason? The research indicates that regardless of why people are gay, their orientation is something that is an integral part of their total selves.

REFERENCES

Hyde, J. S., & DeLamater, J. D. (2008). *Understanding human sexuality* (10th ed.). New York: McGraw-Hill.

Chapter 13 Competencies/Practice Behaviors Exercises Assessment:

Name: ______________________________ **Date:** __________
Supervisor's Name: ____________________

Focus Competencies or Practice Behaviors:

- EP 2.1.1b Practice personal reflection and self-correction to assure continual professional development
- EP 2.1.2a Recognize and manage personal values in a way that allows professional values to guide practice
- EP 2.1.4a Recognize the extent to which a culture's structures and values may oppress, marginalize, alienate, or create or enhance privilege and power
- EP 2.1.4b Gain sufficient self-awareness to eliminate the influence of personal biases and values in working with diverse groups
- EP 2.1.4c Recognize and communicate their understanding of the importance of difference in shaping life experiences
- EP 2.1.5a Understand forms and mechanisms of oppression and discrimination
- EP 2.1.5b Advocate for human rights and social and economic justice

Instructions:

A. Evaluate your work or your partner's work in the Focus Competencies/Practice Behaviors by completing the Competencies/Practice Behaviors Assessment form below

B. What other Competencies/Practice Behaviors did you use to complete these Exercises? Be sure to record them in your assessments

1.	I have attained this competency/practice behavior (in the range of 81 to 100%)
2.	I have largely attained this competency/practice behavior (in the range of 61 to 80%)
3.	I have partially attained this competency/practice behavior (in the range of 41 to 60%)
4.	I have made a little progress in attaining this competency/practice behavior (in the range of 21 to 40%)
5.	I have made almost no progress in attaining this competency/practice behavior (in the range of 0 to 20%)

EPAS 2008 Core Competencies & Core Practice Behaviors	Student Self Assessment						Evaluator Feedback
Student and Evaluator Assessment Scale and Comments	**0**	**1**	**2**	**3**	**4**	**5**	**Agree/Disagree/Comments**
EP 2.1.1 Identify as a Professional Social Worker and Conduct Oneself Accordingly:							
a. Advocate for client access to the services of social work							
b. Practice personal reflection and self-correction to assure continual professional development							
c. Attend to professional roles and boundaries							
d. Demonstrate professional demeanor in behavior, appearance, and communication							
e. Engage in career-long learning							
f. Use supervision and consultation							

EP 2.1.2 Apply Social Work Ethical Principles to Guide Professional Practice:								
a.	Recognize and manage personal values in a way that allows professional values to guide practice							
b.	Make ethical decisions by applying NASW Code of Ethics and, as applicable, of the IFSW/IASSW Ethics in Social Work, Statement of Principles							
c.	Tolerate ambiguity in resolving ethical conflicts							
d.	Apply strategies of ethical reasoning to arrive at principled decisions							
EP 2.1.3 Apply Critical Thinking to Inform and Communicate Professional Judgments:								
a.	Distinguish, appraise, and integrate multiple sources of knowledge, including research-based knowledge and practice wisdom							
b.	Analyze models of assessment, prevention, intervention, and evaluation							
c.	Demonstrate effective oral and written communication in working with individuals, families, groups, organizations, communities, and colleagues							
EP 2.1.4 Engage Diversity and Difference in Practice:								
a.	Recognize the extent to which a culture's structures and values may oppress, marginalize, alienate, or create or enhance privilege and power							
b.	Gain sufficient self-awareness to eliminate the influence of personal biases and values in working with diverse groups							
c.	Recognize and communicate their understanding of the importance of difference in shaping life experiences							
d.	View themselves as learners and engage those with whom they work as informants							
EP 2.1.5 Advance Human Rights and Social and Economic Justice:								
a.	Understand forms and mechanisms of oppression and discrimination							
b.	Advocate for human rights and social and economic justice							
c.	Engage in practices that advance social and economic justice							
EP 2.1.6 Engage in Research-Informed Practice and Practice-Informed Research:								
a.	Use practice experience to inform scientific inquiry							
b.	Use research evidence to inform practice							
EP 2.1.7 Apply Knowledge of Human Behavior and the Social Environment:								
a.	Utilize conceptual frameworks to guide the processes of assessment, intervention, and evaluation							
b.	Critique and apply knowledge to understand person and environment							

EP 2.1.8 Engage in Policy Practice to Advance Social and Economic Well-Being and to Deliver Effective Social Work Services:								
a.	Analyze, formulate, and advocate for policies that advance social well-being							
b.	Collaborate with colleagues and clients for effective policy action							
EP 2.1.9 Respond to Contexts that Shape Practice:								
a.	Continuously discover, appraise, and attend to changing locales, populations, scientific and technological developments, and emerging societal trends to provide relevant services							
b.	Provide leadership in promoting sustainable changes in service delivery and practice to improve the quality of social services							
EP 2.1.10 Engage, Assess, Intervene, and Evaluate with Individuals, Families, Groups, Organizations and Communities:								
a.	Substantively and affectively prepare for action with individuals, families, groups, organizations, and communities							
b.	Use empathy and other interpersonal skills							
c.	Develop a mutually agreed-on focus of work and desired outcomes							
d.	Collect, organize, and interpret client data							
e.	Assess client strengths and limitations							
f.	Develop mutually agreed-on intervention goals and objectives							
g.	Select appropriate intervention strategies							
h.	Initiate actions to achieve organizational goals							
i.	Implement prevention interventions that enhance client capacities							
j.	Help clients resolve problems							
k.	Negotiate, mediate, and advocate for clients							
l.	Facilitate transitions and endings							
m.	Critically analyze, monitor, and evaluate interventions							

Chapter 14
Biological Aspects of Later Adulthood

Competencies/Practice Behaviors Exercise 14.1
Later Adulthood Can Be Rewarding

Focus Competencies or Practice Behaviors:

- EP 2.1.3a Distinguish, appraise, and integrate multiple sources of knowledge, including research-based knowledge and practice wisdom
- EP 2.1.7b Critique and apply knowledge to understand person and environment

A. Brief description
You will contact an older person to gather information, which is then shared in class.

B. Objectives
You will:
1. Have a greater appreciation that later adulthood can be enjoyable and rewarding.
2. Identify factors that contribute to good physical and mental health.

C. Procedure
1. Talk to an older friend or relative who appears to be enjoying life and who is in fairly good health. (If you cannot meet with this person, telephone him or her.) Ask (a) what activities make this person's life enjoyable, and (b) to what does he or she attribute his or her good health?
2. At the designated class period, form subgroups of four or five persons. Describe positive qualities and characteristics of the person you talked to and then summarize their responses to the questions.
3. A representative of each group presents a summary of activities that make the respondents' lives enjoyable and to what they attribute their good health.
4. Discuss the consistency between the chapter presentation of factors that promote good health and those mentioned by the respondents.

Competencies/Practice Behaviors Exercise 14.2
Interviewing an Older Person Role-Play

Focus Competencies or Practice Behaviors:

- EP 2.1.1b Practice personal reflection and self-correction to assure continual professional development
- EP 2.1.3a Distinguish, appraise, and integrate multiple sources of knowledge, including research-based knowledge and practice wisdom
- EP 2.1.7b Critique and apply knowledge to understand person and environment

A. Brief description
The instructor asks for a volunteer (for which extra credit is given) to invite and interview in class an older person who is still active and who has had interesting life experiences.

B. Objectives

You will:

1. Gain an appreciation of what it is like to be an older person in our society.
2. Be motivated to have more contact and communication with the older persons who are relatives, friends, and acquaintances.

C. Procedure

1. Suggested questions for the volunteer to ask the older person follow. The volunteer should follow up on comments, probe as necessary, and ask for clarification. The other students in the class should also be encouraged to ask questions.

QUESTIONS

1. How old are you and where were you born?
2. What did you do for a living? (Can include housewife and mother.)
3. How old do you feel—younger than your age, older?
4. What are your plans for the coming months and years—what would you like to do, accomplish?
5. Would you still like to learn something entirely new—a new job, hobby, or something you always wanted to learn about?
6. In looking back on life, what are some things you feel you've learned that younger people should know about? (Give a few minutes or seconds to think here.)
7. Are there things you'd like to go back and do over again?
8. About friends and family—what have you learned about relationships that are important?
9. What are your views as to the major social problems confronting older people in our society?
10. What are your most memorable high points and low points in life.
11. Do you think you "grew up" in the manner that your parents hoped? That is, do you think your parents would be satisfied with how you turned out? Why or why not?
12. If you could advise me about "life," what's the most important thing you could say to me at my age?

2. When the interview ends, the volunteer should thank the older person.
3. At some later class session, the instructor may ask for another volunteer to invite and interview a different older person.

Competencies/Practice Behaviors Exercise 14.3
Meditation

Focus Competencies or Practice Behaviors:

- EP 2.1.1b Practice personal reflection and self-correction to assure continual professional development
- EP 2.1.7a Utilize conceptual frameworks to guide the processes of assessment, intervention, and evaluation
- EP 2.1.7b Critique and apply knowledge to understand person and environment

A. Brief description
The instructor will lead you in three forms of meditation.

B. Objectives
You will:
1. Experience the enjoyable effects of being deeply relaxed.
2. Learn to describe the harmful effects of stress, and to identify when you are experiencing high levels of stress.
3. Be able to use one or more of these meditative techniques in the future in order to relax when stress levels mount.

C. Procedure
1. Using the material in the chapter, the instructor briefly summarizes what stress is and indicates that prolonged high levels of stress lead to emotional disorders, behavioral disorders, and stress-related illnesses. It is important for each person to learn some ways to reduce stress.
2. Many people are unaware of moderately elevated levels of stress. By becoming more conscious of your body signals, you can learn to identify when stress levels are too high. Look at the section below, "Signals for a Good Level of Stress and for A Too High a Level of Stress." With practice you can learn awareness of body signals that indicate when levels of stress are too high.

SIGNALS FOR A GOOD LEVEL OF STRESS AND FOR A TOO-HIGH LEVEL OF STRESS

Good Level of Stress	Level of Stress Too High
1. Feelings	
Excitement, exhilaration	Anxiety, fear, timidity
Pleasure, enjoyment	Anger, resentfulness, dissatisfaction, bitterness
Relaxation, calmness	Confusion, feelings of being overwhelmed or swamped
Feeling of confidence	Helplessness or powerlessness
	Fear of inadequacy or failure
	Tension or tightness
	Depression, weariness, feeling fed up
	Paranoia
2. Behaviors	
Smile, laugh, joke	Engage in wasted motion and activity
Act intelligent and knowledgeable	Irritable—put people down
Sensitive to others, appreciate others, and recognize contributions of others	Unpleasant to be around
Get a lot done—productive	Let little things get to you
	Impatient

Able to listen to others Generally successful Friendly Creative; make good decisions	Tend to be easily startled by small sounds Unable to concentrate Stutter Smoke to excess Overeat or overdrink (e.g., coffee) Poor work quality Not creative High-pitched nervous laughter

3. Body Reactions

Coordinated body reactions Absence of ill health Absence of aches and pains Unaware of your body, which functions smoothly Sleep soundly	Various aches and pains in head, muscles, back, neck Ulcers or upset stomach Sleep problems Skin rashes, itches, skin irritations Breathing irregularities or asthma Tense or tight muscles High blood pressure Frequent colds, flu Feelings of weakness or dizziness Trembling, nervous tics Sweating, frequent need to urinate Diarrhea or vomiting; loss of appetite; accident prone

3. Learning to meditate is one way to reduce stress. The instructor leads you in three meditative exercises. The purpose is to demonstrate that through meditating you can become deeply relaxed. You can do these exercises by yourself, whenever you are anxious and want to relax. For example, you can use them to relax prior to taking an important exam or giving a speech. You may also want to do these exercises before going to bed at night in order to fall asleep faster. The instructor slowly reads the following to the class, pausing occasionally. (The instructor is free to modify what is said to the class.)

Herbert Benson, who wrote *The Relaxation Response*, has identified four key elements common to meditative approaches that help people to relax. These four elements are: (1) being in a quiet place; (2) getting in a comfortable position; (3) having an object to dwell on, such as your breathing, or thinking about your ideal relaxation place, or a neutral word or phrase that you continually repeat silently; and (4) having a passive attitude in which you let go of your day-to-day concerns by no longer thinking about them. Having a passive attitude is the key element in helping you to relax.

Now, I want you to form a circle. [Wait until a circle is formed.] I will lead you in three types of meditation. First, we will do a deep breathing exercise. Then, we will repeat the word "Relax" silently to ourselves. Third, I'll have you focus on visualizing your most relaxing place. We will move directly from the first to the second, and then from the second to the third without stopping. When we do this exercise, don't worry about anything unusual happening. There will be no tricks. Concentrate on what I'm telling you to focus on, while taking a passive attitude where you let go of your everyday thoughts and concerns. Everyday thoughts and concerns may occasionally enter your mind, but seek to let go of them when they do.

Before we start, I want each of you to identify one of your most relaxing scenes. It may be lying in the sun on a beach or by a lake. It may be sitting in warm water in a bathtub reading a book. It may be sitting by a warm fireplace. Is there anyone who hasn't identified a relaxing scene? [Wait until everyone has identified one.]

OK, we're ready to start. [If possible, dim the lights, or turn out some of them.] First, I want you to close your eyes and keep them closed for the entire exercise. Next, get in a comfortable position. If you want, you can sit or lie on the floor. [Take five or six minutes for each of the three meditative exercises. Speak softly and slowly. Pause frequently, sometimes for twenty seconds or more without saying anything. Feel free to add material to the following instructions.]

First, I want you to focus only on your breathing. Breathe in and out slowly and deeply...Breathe in and out slowly...as you breathe out feel how relaxing it feels...While exhaling, imagine your concerns are leaving you...as you're breathing in and out, feel how you're becoming more calm, more relaxed, more refreshed...Just keep focusing on breathing slowly in and out...Don't try to be in sync when I'm talking about breathing in and out...Find a breathing rhythm that's comfortable for you...Breathe in slowly and deeply, and then slowly breathe out...You've got the power within you to get more and more relaxed...All you have to do is focus on your breathing...Breathe in slowly and deeply, and then slowly breathe out...If other thoughts happen to enter your mind, just let them drift away as effortlessly as possible...The key to becoming more relaxed is to let go of your day-to-day concerns...To do this, all you need to do is simply focus on your breathing...Breathe in slowly and deeply, and then breathe out.

Now we will switch to repeating silently to yourself the word "Relax." Keep your eyes closed...just keep repeating to yourself the word "Relax"...Keep repeating "Relax" to yourself silently and slowly...If day-to-day thoughts enter your mind, seek to stop thinking about them...Keep repeating "Relax" to yourself...All of us encounter daily stressors...It is impossible to avoid daily stressors...The important thing to remember about stress management is not to seek to avoid daily stressors but to find ways to relax when we are under high levels of stress...An excellent and very simple way to learn to relax is to sit in a quiet place, in a comfortable position, and silently repeat to yourself the word "Relax"... "Relax" ... "Relax"...By simply repeating the word "Relax" to yourself, you have the power within you to become more and more relaxed...Find a nice comfortable pace for repeating the word "Relax" to yourself...The pace should be slow enough so that you can relax...But not be so slow that thoughts about your day-to-day concerns enter your mind...Remember, the key to relaxing is letting go of your day-to-day concerns...If such concerns begin to enter your mind, focus more of your attention on repeating "Relax" silently and slowly to yourself...By repeating "Relax" to yourself, you will find it will appear to have magical powers for you, as you will find yourself becoming more and more relaxed and refreshed...[Have the members repeat "Relax" for five or six minutes.]

Now, we will switch to focusing on your most relaxing scene. Don't open your eyes...Focus on being in your most relaxing place...Feel how good and relaxing it feels...Just dwell on how relaxing it feels...Enjoy everything about how calm and relaxing this place is...Feel yourself becoming calmer, more relaxed...Enjoy the peacefulness of this place...Feel yourself becoming more relaxed, more renewed and refreshed...Enjoy all the sights and sounds of this special place for you...Notice and cherish the pleasant smells and aromas...Feel the warmth, peacefulness, and serenity of this very special place for you... Whenever you want to become more relaxed, all you have to do is close your eyes, sit quietly, and visualize yourself being in this very relaxing place...The more you practice visualizing being in your relaxing place, the quicker you will find yourself becoming relaxed...It will appear to you that your relaxing place has magical, relaxing powers for you, but in reality you are simply relaxing yourself by letting go of your day-to-day concerns and instead focusing on enjoying the peacefulness of your most relaxing place...If you have to give a speech, or are facing some other stressful situation, you can learn to reduce your level of anxiety by simply closing your eyes for a short period of time and focusing your thoughts on being in your most relaxing place... You always have the power within you to reduce your level of anxiety...All you have to do is close your eyes and visualize being in your very special relaxing place...Continue to visualize, now, being in this very relaxing place...Feel yourself becoming more relaxed, refreshed, and calm...If you're feeling drowsy, that's fine...Feeling drowsy is an indication that you're becoming more and more relaxed...You're doing fine...Just keep on visualizing being in your very relaxing place...You will become more and more relaxed by simply letting go of your day-to-day concerns and by enjoying this very special relaxing place...[Pause, then continue this exercise for five or six minutes.]

Unfortunately, in a minute or so, it will be time to return to this class, but there is no hurry. I will slowly count backward from 5 to 1, and then ask you to open your eyes shortly after we reach 1... 5. Enjoy how relaxed you feel. You may now feel warmer, drowsy, and so relaxed that you feel you don't even want to move a muscle...Enjoy this very special feeling...It is so healthy to become this relaxed as your immune system functions best when you are relaxed... 4. Slowly begin to return to this class...There is no rush...There is no hurry...Take your time to become more alert. Anytime you want to relax, all you need to do is use one of these three meditative approaches. With practice, you will gradually get better at relaxing by using these approaches... 3. You should now focus on returning in a short time to this class...Take your time...We still have a half-minute or so...Examine whether you want to make a commitment to use relaxation exercises to reduce the daily stress you encounter... 2. We are nearly at the time to return to this class...You should now work toward becoming more and more alert... 1. Slowly open your eyes...There is no hurry...Take your time to get oriented. A word of caution: If you have to drive some place soon, please walk around for several minutes before trying to drive a car, as you may be so relaxed now that you may not be alert enough to drive safely.

4. What do you think of these three approaches? How relaxed did you get? Did you have trouble getting relaxed? If yes, why? Which of the three approaches did you like best and why?

Chapter 14 Competencies/Practice Behaviors Exercises Assessment:

Name: ________________________________ **Date:** __________
Supervisor's Name: ________________________________

Focus Competencies/Practice Behaviors:

- EP 2.1.1b Practice personal reflection and self-correction to assure continual professional development
- EP 2.1.3c Demonstrate effective oral and written communication in working with individuals, families, groups, organizations, communities, and colleagues
- EP 2.1.4b Gain sufficient self-awareness to eliminate the influence of personal biases and values in working with diverse groups
- EP 2.1.4c Recognize and communicate their understanding of the importance of difference in shaping life experiences
- EP 2.1.7a Utilize conceptual frameworks to guide the processes of assessment, intervention, and evaluation
- EP 2.1.10a Substantively and affectively prepare for action with individuals, families, groups, organizations, and communities
- EP 2.1.10b Use empathy and other interpersonal skills
- EP 2.1.10d Collect, organize, and interpret client data
- EP 2.1.10e Assess client strengths and limitations

Instructions:

A. Evaluate your work or your partner's work in the Focus Competencies/Practice Behaviors by completing the Competencies/Practice Behaviors Assessment form below

B. What other Competencies/Practice Behaviors did you use to complete these Exercises? Be sure to record them in your assessments

1.	I have attained this competency/practice behavior (in the range of 81 to 100%)
2.	I have largely attained this competency/practice behavior (in the range of 61 to 80%)
3.	I have partially attained this competency/practice behavior (in the range of 41 to 60%)
4.	I have made a little progress in attaining this competency/practice behavior (in the range of 21 to 40%)
5.	I have made almost no progress in attaining this competency/practice behavior (in the range of 0 to 20%)

EPAS 2008 Core Competencies & Core Practice Behaviors	Student Self Assessment						Evaluator Feedback
Student and Evaluator Assessment Scale and Comments	0	1	2	3	4	5	Agree/Disagree/Comments
EP 2.1.1 Identify as a Professional Social Worker and Conduct Oneself Accordingly:							
a. Advocate for client access to the services of social work							
b. Practice personal reflection and self-correction to assure continual professional development							
c. Attend to professional roles and boundaries							
d. Demonstrate professional demeanor in behavior, appearance, and communication							

e. Engage in career-long learning							
f. Use supervision and consultation							
EP 2.1.2 Apply Social Work Ethical Principles to Guide Professional Practice:							
a. Recognize and manage personal values in a way that allows professional values to guide practice							
b. Make ethical decisions by applying NASW Code of Ethics and, as applicable, of the IFSW/IASSW Ethics in Social Work, Statement of Principles							
c. Tolerate ambiguity in resolving ethical conflicts							
d. Apply strategies of ethical reasoning to arrive at principled decisions							
EP 2.1.3 Apply Critical Thinking to Inform and Communicate Professional Judgments:							
a. Distinguish, appraise, and integrate multiple sources of knowledge, including research-based knowledge and practice wisdom							
b. Analyze models of assessment, prevention, intervention, and evaluation							
c. Demonstrate effective oral and written communication in working with individuals, families, groups, organizations, communities, and colleagues							
EP 2.1.4 Engage Diversity and Difference in Practice:							
a. Recognize the extent to which a culture's structures and values may oppress, marginalize, alienate, or create or enhance privilege and power							
b. Gain sufficient self-awareness to eliminate the influence of personal biases and values in working with diverse groups							
c. Recognize and communicate their understanding of the importance of difference in shaping life experiences							
d. View themselves as learners and engage those with whom they work as informants							
EP 2.1.5 Advance Human Rights and Social and Economic Justice:							
a. Understand forms and mechanisms of oppression and discrimination							
b. Advocate for human rights and social and economic justice							
c. Engage in practices that advance social and economic justice							
EP 2.1.6 Engage in Research-Informed Practice and Practice-Informed Research:							
a. Use practice experience to inform scientific inquiry							
b. Use research evidence to inform practice							
EP 2.1.7 Apply Knowledge of Human Behavior and the Social Environment:							
a. Utilize conceptual frameworks to guide the processes of assessment, intervention, and evaluation							
b. Critique and apply knowledge to understand person and environment							

EP 2.1.8 Engage in Policy Practice to Advance Social and Economic Well-Being and to Deliver Effective Social Work Services:							
a. Analyze, formulate, and advocate for policies that advance social well-being							
b. Collaborate with colleagues and clients for effective policy action							
EP 2.1.9 Respond to Contexts that Shape Practice:							
a. Continuously discover, appraise, and attend to changing locales, populations, scientific and technological developments, and emerging societal trends to provide relevant services							
b. Provide leadership in promoting sustainable changes in service delivery and practice to improve the quality of social services							
EP 2.1.10 Engage, Assess, Intervene, and Evaluate with Individuals, Families, Groups, Organizations and Communities:							
a. Substantively and affectively prepare for action with individuals, families, groups, organizations, and communities							
b. Use empathy and other interpersonal skills							
c. Develop a mutually agreed-on focus of work and desired outcomes							
d. Collect, organize, and interpret client data							
e. Assess client strengths and limitations							
f. Develop mutually agreed-on intervention goals and objectives							
g. Select appropriate intervention strategies							
h. Initiate actions to achieve organizational goals							
i. Implement prevention interventions that enhance client capacities							
j. Help clients resolve problems							
k. Negotiate, mediate, and advocate for clients							
l. Facilitate transitions and endings							
m. Critically analyze, monitor, and evaluate interventions							

Chapter 15
Psychological Aspects of Later Adulthood

Competencies/Practice Behaviors Exercise 15.1
Attitudes Toward Later Adulthood

Focus Competencies or Practice Behaviors:

- EP 2.1.1b Practice personal reflection and self-correction to assure continual professional development
- EP 2.1.6b Use research evidence to inform practice
- EP 2.1.7a Utilize conceptual frameworks to guide the processes of assessment, intervention, and evaluation
- EP 2.1.7b Critique and apply knowledge to understand person and environment
- EP 2.1.8a Analyze, formulate, and advocate for policies that advance social well-being

A. Brief description
You will complete an attitudinal questionnaire about later adulthood, and the responses will be discussed.

B. Objectives
You will:
1. Be more aware of your attitudes toward and values concerning later adulthood.
2. Be able to identify prejudicial statements about older people.

C. Procedure
1. Answer the following ten questions related to your attitudes about later adulthood. Write your answers on a sheet of paper or a five-by-seven-inch notecard. Do not write your name on the response sheet.
2. The instructor will slowly read the following questions, giving you time to record your responses. Alternatively, you may read the questions from this manual.

a. Do you currently have a friend or relative over age 65 with whom you frequently discuss your concerns?
____ Yes ____ No

b. Do you believe that most people over age 65 are physically attractive?
____ Yes ____ No

c. Do you believe that it is desirable for older people to be sexually active?
____ Yes ____ No

d. Do you want to spend the last few years of your life in a nursing home?
____ Yes ____ No

e. Are you looking forward to being over age 65?
____ Yes ____ No

f. If one of your parents should die, would you want your other parent to remarry?
____ Yes ____ No

g. If an older person had a terminal illness, was in severe pain, and had no hope of a recovery, do you think it would be appropriate for this person to terminate his or her life by suicide?
____ Yes ____ No

h. Do you believe that an older person should be forced to retire when they reach a certain age, such as age 70?
____ Yes ____ No

i. How old would you like to be when you die?
____ Age

j. If an older person has a terminal illness and is in a coma, should that person be kept alive by life-sustaining equipment?
____ Yes ____ No

3. The instructor collects the responses and lists the letter of each question on the chalkboard, from (a) through (j). Volunteers record the responses.
4. Reread each question, and discuss the responses.

Competencies/Practice Behaviors Exercise 15.2
Learning to Grieve Constructively

Focus Competencies or Practice Behaviors:

- EP 2.1.1b Practice personal reflection and self-correction to assure continual professional development
- EP 2.1.3a Distinguish, appraise, and integrate multiple sources of knowledge, including research-based knowledge and practice wisdom
- EP 2.1.3b Analyze models of assessment, prevention, intervention, and evaluation
- EP 2.1.7a Utilize conceptual frameworks to guide the processes of assessment, intervention, and evaluation
- EP 2.1.7b Critique and apply knowledge to understand person and environment

A. Brief description
Through a visualization exercise, you will review how you handle a significant loss. Volunteers will share their grieving experiences. Suggestions are given on how to handle significant losses constructively.

B. Objectives
You will:
1. Understand two models of the grieving process.
2. Be able to more effectively handle past, present, and future losses.

C. Procedure

1. The instructor summarizes the Kübler-Ross and Westberg models of the grieving process. (As an alternative, you can read this material in the text.)
2. This exercise is designed to help you get in touch with a grief experience that you have had. The exercise may become intense. If it becomes too intense, it is certainly acceptable if you leave the room temporarily.
3. The instructor asks you (and the other students) to close your eyes. There will be no surprises in this exercise. The instructor reads the following slowly, pausing frequently:

First, I want to have you get as relaxed and comfortable as possible...Take several deep breaths, while breathing in and out slowly...I want you now to focus on the greatest loss you have experienced...It might be the death of someone close to you...It might be the end of a romantic relationship...It might be moving away from friends and family...It might be the death of a pet...It might be not getting as high a grade on a test or in a course that you had hoped for...Whatever it is, concentrate on it...

When you were first informed about the loss, were you in a state of shock?...Did you deny the loss?...Were you, at times, angry about the loss?...Did you, at times, seek to bargain about the loss?...If you did seek to bargain, whom did you seek to bargain with?...Were you, at times, depressed about the loss?...If you were depressed, why (specifically) were you depressed?...Did you at times have some fears or concerns about the loss?...If you had fears or concerns, what were these fears or concerns?...Did you at times have guilt about this loss?...If you did feel guilty, what specifically did you feel guilty about? Did you cry about this loss?...If you cried, do you know why you cried?...If you didn't cry, do you know why you didn't cry?...If you cried, was it helpful?...How deeply has this loss hurt you?...How long have you been hurting about this loss?...

Do you at times still grieve deeply about this loss?...Have you found that as time goes on you are grieving less deeply, and that your intense grieving periods are shorter in duration?...Do holidays, anniversaries, birthdays, special days still remind you of the loss?...If and when you are grieving deeply, how do you seek to handle this grief?...

Has the loss been so great that you thought about taking your life?...Many people think about taking their life when they are grieving deeply...Have you made attempts to take your life?...

Have you had some physical reactions to the loss, such as difficulty in sleeping, stomach problems, headaches, anxiety attacks, sexual difficulties?...Grieving is very stressful, and it is common to have physical reactions...Do you dream about the loss?...For example, it is common for people who have lost a loved one to dream that person is still alive...Often when someone awakes from such a dream, it is difficult to separate reality from the dream...

What aspects of the loss have you handled well?...What aspects could you have handled better?...What aspects are you still working on?...How have you gone about handling this loss?...How pleased are you with your efforts to handle this loss?...How have others close to you handled this loss?...How have you gone about helping them?...Have you grown from this loss experience?...What yet do you need to work on to handle this loss?...What specific efforts are you making to handle this loss?...OK...slowly open your eyes, and let's talk about grieving.

4. The instructor indicates that one of the best ways to handle grief is to talk about it. The instructor asks if someone wishes to share a loss he or she has experienced and describe

what helped him or her to handle this loss. If no one begins to share a grieving experience, the instructor describes a personal loss and how it was handled.

5. The class discusses whether the Westberg model or the Kübler-Ross model of the grieving process can better describe the grief they experienced. The instructor ends the exercise by summarizing material given in the chapter on how to handle grief constructively.

Competencies/Practice Behaviors Exercise 15.3
Becoming Comfortable With Your Own Death

Focus Competencies or Practice Behaviors:

- EP 2.1.1b Practice personal reflection and self-correction to assure continual professional development
- EP 2.1.3a Distinguish, appraise, and integrate multiple sources of knowledge, including research-based knowledge and practice wisdom
- EP 2.1.7b Critique and apply knowledge to understand person and environment

A. Brief description

Through a visualization exercise, reflect on your reactions to being informed that you have a terminal illness. A discussion follows.

B. Objectives

You will:

1. Examine your fears about death and dying.
2. Become sufficiently comfortable with the concept of death so that you will be able to rationally contemplate your own eventual death.

C. Procedure

1. This is a visualization exercise. The instructor reads the following slowly:

> I want you to close your eyes and get as comfortable as possible. Take several deep breaths, while breathing in and out slowly. There will be no surprises in this exercise. (pause) Imagine that you haven't been feeling well for a period of time, and that you go to your doctor for a series of tests. The tests are taken, and you have an appointment to be informed about the results. The doctor has a concerned look and asks you to be seated. The doctor informs you that you have a terminal illness and estimates that you have about six or seven months to live. Does this scene seem believable? I know this scene may be difficult for some of you to imagine, as many of us like to think we will live for a very long time and don't want to think about our own death. If we are to become comfortable with our own death, we need to think about it and prepare for it. One way of doing so is through an exercise like this. Therefore, I ask you to concentrate as fully as you can on this scene in which you have just been informed you have a terminal illness.
>
> What are you thinking and feeling? Are you in a state of shock? Are you actively denying that this could happen? Are you breathing faster? Are your eyes watering? Is your heart beating faster? Are you numbed by this? Are you terrified? Do you have fears about the pain you may experience in your remaining months?

What do you want to do? Are you interested in seeking more information about your illness from your physician? Do you want to leave the office? When you leave the office, what do you want to do—drive home? Tell friends or relatives? Be by yourself? What do you plan to do with the remaining months you have left to live? Do you want to travel? Would you seek to change your lifestyle? Would you seek to satisfy hedonistic desires such as sex or drugs? Would you become more withdrawn? Would you become more religious and pray more? Would you seek to complete projects and tie up loose ends? Would you become concerned about preparing dependents and friends about your death? Would you consider committing suicide?

If it were possible, would you want to know the exact date on which you will die? What efforts do you believe ought to be made to keep you alive? All possible medical efforts even though there is no hope of returning to a quality life? Or, would you want medical efforts to be discontinued when there is little hope to return to a quality life?

What aspect of your own death is most distasteful to you? Is it that you will no longer have enjoyable experiences? Is it that you are afraid of what will happen to your body and mind after you die? Is it that you are uncertain as to what might happen to you if there is a life after death? Are you worried about what will happen to people who depend upon you? Are you concerned that your plans and projects might come to an end? Are you worried about your relatives and friends grieving about you? Are you worried about the pain you may experience before you die? Are you worried that your body may deteriorate as you die?

How would you want people to remember you? What would you like placed on your tombstone? If you want people to remember you in a certain way, are you living your life in such a way that they will remember you as you desire?

What kind of funeral do you want? Do you want a lot of people at your funeral? Or, do you want only close relatives and friends to be at your funeral? Do you want a church service? Do you want a lot of flowers at your funeral? Is there a certain song that you wish would be played? Do you think funerals are primarily for those who died, or for survivors to help them cope with the loss? Do you want a burial, or do you wish to be cremated? Have you considered donating parts of your body for organ transplants? Have you considered donating your body to a medical school or to science? If mystery surrounded your death, would you want an autopsy?

What does death mean to you? How is what happens after you die different from what life was like before you were born? Do you view death as the absolute end of life? Do you view death as being a transition to a new life? Do you view death as being a joining of your spirit with a cosmic force? Do you view death as being an endless sleep? Do you view death as the termination of this life, but with the survival of your spirit or soul? Do you believe that there is an afterlife?

If you would want to make changes in your life upon learning you have a terminal illness, what is preventing you from making these changes at the present time? OK, slowly open your eyes and let's talk.

2. The instructor discusses the exercise with the class, including the following questions:
   a. Did you have trouble visualizing the exercise as being real?
   b. If so, why do you think you had trouble?
   c. Do you think the exercise was helpful in getting you to think about, and become comfortable with, your eventual death?

Competencies/Practice Behaviors Exercise 15.4
An Epitaph as a Guide to Living

Focus Competencies or Practice Behaviors:

- EP 2.1.1b Practice personal reflection and self-correction to assure continual professional development

A. Brief description

You will write an epitaph that is anonymously shared with the class.

B. Objectives

You will:

1. Better accept your eventual death.
2. Specify a broad-based statement as to how you want to live life prior to dying.
3. Compare your "guide to living" with that of others.

C. Procedure

1. A sheet of paper or a large notecard is distributed to each of you. Write down the epitaph you want placed on your tombstone. An epitaph is a brief statement or phrase describing the deceased. Do not put your name on the paper.
2. The instructor collects the epitaphs in a way that prevents them from being identified and reads them to the class.

Competencies/Practice Behaviors Exercise 15.5
Questions About Grief, Death, and Dying

Focus Competencies or Practice Behaviors:

- EP 2.1.1b Practice personal reflection and self-correction to assure continual professional development
- EP 2.1.7a Utilize conceptual frameworks to guide the processes of assessment, intervention, and evaluation
- EP 2.1.7b Critique and apply knowledge to understand person and environment

A. Brief description

You are asked to complete a questionnaire that forces you to confront personal feelings about death.

B. Objectives

You will:

1. Examine your personal feelings about death.
2. Increase your ability to empathize with persons who are coping with their own death or the death of a loved one.

C. Procedure

1. Fill out the following questionnaire:

QUESTIONS ABOUT GRIEF, DEATH, AND DYING

(For the multiple-choice questions, circle all of the items that apply to you)

1. Which of the following describe your present conception of death:
   a. Cessation of all mental and physical activity
   b. Sleep
   c. Existence in heaven or hell
   d. A pleasant afterlife
   e. Mysterious and unknown
   f. The end of all life
   g. A transition to a new beginning
   h. A joining of the spirit with an unknown cosmic force
   i. Termination of this physical life with survival of the spirit
   j. Something other than the above

2. Which of the following aspects of your own death do you find distasteful:
   a. What might happen to your body after death
   b. What might happen to you if there is a life after death
   c. What might happen to your dependents
   d. The grief that it would cause to your friends and relatives
   e. The pain you may experience as you die
   f. The deterioration of your body before you die
   g. All your plans and projects coming to an end
   h. Something other than the above

3. If you could choose, what age would you like to be when you die?

4. When you think of your own eventual death, how do you feel?
   a. Depressed
   b. Fearful
   c. Discouraged
   d. Purposeless
   e. Angry
   f. Pleasure in being alive
   g. Resigned, as you realize death is a natural process of living
   h. Other (specify)

5. For what, or for whom, would you be willing to sacrifice your life:
   a. An idea or moral principle
   b. A loved one
   c. The nation
   d. An emergency where another life could be saved
   e. Not for any reason

6. If you could choose, how would you prefer to die?
   a. A sudden violent death
   b. A sudden but nonviolent death
   c. A quiet and dignified death
   d. Death in the line of duty
   e. Suicide
   f. Homicide
   g. Death after you have achieved your life goals
   h. Other (specify)

7. If it were possible, would you want to know the exact date on which you would die?

8. Would you want to know if you had a terminal illness?

9. If you had six more months to live, how would you want to spend this time?
   a. Satisfying hedonistic desires such as sex
   b. Withdrawing
   c. Contemplating or praying
   d. Seeking to prepare loved ones for my death
   e. Completing projects and tying up loose ends
   f. Considering suicide
   g. Other (specify)

10. Have you seriously contemplated suicide? What are your moral views of suicide? Are there circumstances under which you would take your life?

11. If you had a serious illness, and the quality of your life had substantially deteriorated, what measures do you believe should be taken to keep you alive?
   a. All possible heroic medical efforts
   b. Medical efforts being discontinued when there is practically no hope of returning to a life with quality
   c. Other (specify)

12. If you are married, would you prefer to outlive your spouse? Why?

13. How important do you believe funerals and grief rituals are for survivors?

14. If it were up to you, how would you like to have your body disposed of after you die?
   a. Cremation
   b. Burial
   c. Donation of body parts for organ transplants
   d. Donation of body to medical school or to science
   e. Other (specify)

15. What kind of funeral would you prefer?
   a. A church service
   b. As large as possible
   c. Small with only close friends and relatives present
   d. A lavish funeral
   e. A simple funeral
   f. Whatever survivors want
   g. Other (specify)

16. Have you made a will? Why or why not?

17. Have you signed a living will? Why or why not?

18. Were you able to arrive at answers to most of these questions? Were you uncomfortable in answering these questions? If you were uncomfortable, what were you feeling, and what made you uncomfortable? For the questions you do not have answers to, how might you arrive at answers?

Competencies/Practice Behaviors Exercise 15.6
Recognizing Life is Terminal

Focus Competencies or Practice Behaviors:

- EP 2.1.1b Practice personal reflection and self-correction to assure continual professional development
- EP 2.1.7b Critique and apply knowledge to understand person and environment

A. Brief description
Through giving up items you deeply cherish, you experience in simulated form feelings related to your own eventual death.

B. Objectives
You will:
1. Become more aware of the thoughts and feelings you will have when your own death becomes imminent.
2. Recognize life is terminal.

C. Procedure

1. The instructor begins by stating that many people do not like to attend funerals, nor do they like to think about their own eventual death. Many people avoid thinking about their own death—they have the irrational notion that their eventual death is so far in the future that they live like they think they will live indefinitely. Yet, grief management authorities assert we need to come to terms with our own death, and that our daily lives will be more meaningful if we become more comfortable with the fact that life is terminal from birth—as we will all die. The instructor then states the objectives of this exercise.
2. The instructor distributes to each student a packet of twelve slips of paper. The students are instructed to write on each of the small slips of paper, one of the following twelve items:

   - Three personal characteristics she is proud of.
   - Three activities she enjoys participating in.
   - The three possessions that she cherishes the most.
   - The names of the three people that are the most important in her life.

   Each student then arranges these twelve slips of paper in front of her on a desk or table so that she can see them all.
3. The instructor states the following: Imagine that you haven't been feeling well for the past several months. You finally decide to see your doctor. The doctor administers a number of medical tests. Today is the day you go in to hear the results of the tests. As you walk in, the doctor has a very concerned look on her face. The doctor informs you that you have a terminal illness. You have thirty seconds to tear up three of your slips of paper.
4. The instructor states the following: You leave the physician's office in a state of shock. You return home. Who is there to greet you? Who do you really want to be there to greet you? What do you say to these people? What do you want to hear from them? Tear up another three slips of paper.
5. The instructor states the following: It is now two months later. You realize your health is deteriorating. Your symptoms are worsening and you are feeling weaker. Where are you now living? Have you made changes in your lifestyle? Are there projects and loose ends in your life that you are seeking to complete? What are you thinking and feeling about your terminal illness? Tear up another two slips of paper.
6. The instructor states the following: It is now four months after you were informed you have a terminal illness. You are undeniably ill. You are in considerable pain, and you now need caregivers to stay alive. Where are you now living? Who is taking care of you? Who visits you? Who are the people you want to visit you and take care of you? Tear up another two slips of paper.
7. The instructor states the following: Six months have now passed since you learned you have a terminal illness. You have very little energy left. The smallest activity of daily living takes most of your energy. A caregiver now has to attend to you 24 hours each day. You no longer can bathe yourself alone. How do you now feel about yourself? Where are you now living? Please turn over your remaining two slips of paper, and I will take one. (The instructor takes one from each student.)
8. The instructor states the following: Look at your last slip of paper, and then tear it up. You are now dead.

9. The instructor thanks the students for conscientiously participating in the first part of this exercise. The instructor then asks the students to form subgroups of about three persons. The members of each subgroup are asked to share their reactions to the following questions, which should now be listed on the blackboard. (If a student chooses not to share, that is his or her personal right.)
   a. Did the exercise seem real? If "yes," when did it become real? If "no," why didn't it seem real?
   b. What emotional reactions did you have to this exercise?
   c. What were the last two items on the slips of paper that you kept?
   d. What were your thoughts, feelings, and reactions to tearing up the last slip of paper?

   The class as a whole then discusses the merits and shortcomings of this exercise.

Competencies/Practice Behaviors Exercise 15.7
Respecting Religious Beliefs Role-Play

Focus Competencies or Practice Behaviors:

- EP 2.1.1b Practice personal reflection and self-correction to assure continual professional development
- EP 2.1.7a Utilize conceptual frameworks to guide the processes of assessment, intervention, and evaluation
- EP 2.1.7b Critique and apply knowledge to understand person and environment

A. Brief description

You will briefly study religions that may differ from your own religious beliefs, and you will examine some religious questions.

B. Objectives

You will:

1. Begin to understand background information about diverse religions.
2. Learn to respect religious beliefs that may differ from your own beliefs.
3. Ultimately make progress in becoming more comfortable with your own religious beliefs.

C. Procedure

1. You first read the boxed material on "spirituality and religion" in the text. This material summarizes background information on Judaism, Christianity, Islam, and Buddhism.
2. You then form subgroups consisting of approximately three students to a group and discuss the following five questions:
   a. Some religions assert that God is all good, all knowing, and all powerful. If God has all three of these characteristics, why would he or she allow diseases like AIDS to occur, or send someone to eternal damnation?
   b. What evidence is there that God existed and that he or she currently exists?
   c. Most of the prominent religions in the world have a "bible," that is, a book of sacred scriptures. Is one of these bibles more accurate in being the word of God than the others? If you answer "yes"—what is it and what evidence do you have?

d. Is there a "one true religion"? If you answer "yes"—what is it and what evidence do you have?

e. If a social worker strongly believes his or her religion is the one true religion, can that worker fully accept clients who are members of some other religious faith?

3. The instructor then asks each subgroup to share its answers with the class. If serious unanswered questions arise during the sharing, the instructor may invite a recognized authority (such as a clergy person or a religious studies professor) to the class to present his or her views on the unanswered questions.
4. The instructor concludes the exercise by asking questions such as the following: Do you believe it is important to respect and understand the religious beliefs of people who hold somewhat different beliefs than what you have? Is intolerance of others' religious beliefs a factor that contributes to other forms of prejudice—such as racism?

Chapter 15 Competencies/Practice Behaviors Exercises Assessment:

Name: ______________________________ **Date:** __________
Supervisor's Name: ____________________

Focus Competencies or Practice Behaviors:

- EP 2.1.1b Practice personal reflection and self-correction to assure continual professional development
- EP 2.1.3a Distinguish, appraise, and integrate multiple sources of knowledge, including research-based knowledge and practice wisdom
- EP 2.1.3b Analyze models of assessment, prevention, intervention, and evaluation
- EP 2.1.6b Use research evidence to inform practice
- EP 2.1.7a Utilize conceptual frameworks to guide the processes of assessment, intervention, and evaluation
- EP 2.1.7b Critique and apply knowledge to understand person and environment
- EP 2.1.8a Analyze, formulate, and advocate for policies that advance social well-being

Instructions:

A. Evaluate your work or your partner's work in the Focus Competencies/Practice Behaviors by completing the Competencies/Practice Behaviors Assessment form below

B. What other Competencies/Practice Behaviors did you use to complete these Exercises? Be sure to record them in your assessments

1.	I have attained this competency/practice behavior (in the range of 81 to 100%)
2.	I have largely attained this competency/practice behavior (in the range of 61 to 80%)
3.	I have partially attained this competency/practice behavior (in the range of 41 to 60%)
4.	I have made a little progress in attaining this competency/practice behavior (in the range of 21 to 40%)
5.	I have made almost no progress in attaining this competency/practice behavior (in the range of 0 to 20%)

EPAS 2008 Core Competencies & Core Practice Behaviors	Student Self Assessment						Evaluator Feedback
Student and Evaluator Assessment Scale and Comments	0	1	2	3	4	5	Agree/Disagree/Comments
EP 2.1.1 Identify as a Professional Social Worker and Conduct Oneself Accordingly:							
a. Advocate for client access to the services of social work							
b. Practice personal reflection and self-correction to assure continual professional development							
c. Attend to professional roles and boundaries							
d. Demonstrate professional demeanor in behavior, appearance, and communication							
e. Engage in career-long learning							
f. Use supervision and consultation							

EP 2.1.2 Apply Social Work Ethical Principles to Guide Professional Practice:							
a. Recognize and manage personal values in a way that allows professional values to guide practice							
b. Make ethical decisions by applying NASW Code of Ethics and, as applicable, of the IFSW/IASSW Ethics in Social Work, Statement of Principles							
c. Tolerate ambiguity in resolving ethical conflicts							
d. Apply strategies of ethical reasoning to arrive at principled decisions							
EP 2.1.3 Apply Critical Thinking to Inform and Communicate Professional Judgments:							
a. Distinguish, appraise, and integrate multiple sources of knowledge, including research-based knowledge and practice wisdom							
b. Analyze models of assessment, prevention, intervention, and evaluation							
c. Demonstrate effective oral and written communication in working with individuals, families, groups, organizations, communities, and colleagues							
EP 2.1.4 Engage Diversity and Difference in Practice:							
a. Recognize the extent to which a culture's structures and values may oppress, marginalize, alienate, or create or enhance privilege and power							
b. Gain sufficient self-awareness to eliminate the influence of personal biases and values in working with diverse groups							
c. Recognize and communicate their understanding of the importance of difference in shaping life experiences							
d. View themselves as learners and engage those with whom they work as informants							
EP 2.1.5 Advance Human Rights and Social and Economic Justice:							
a. Understand forms and mechanisms of oppression and discrimination							
b. Advocate for human rights and social and economic justice							
c. Engage in practices that advance social and economic justice							
EP 2.1.6 Engage in Research-Informed Practice and Practice-Informed Research:							
a. Use practice experience to inform scientific inquiry							
b. Use research evidence to inform practice							
EP 2.1.7 Apply Knowledge of Human Behavior and the Social Environment:							
a. Utilize conceptual frameworks to guide the processes of assessment, intervention, and evaluation							
b. Critique and apply knowledge to understand person and environment							

EP 2.1.8 Engage in Policy Practice to Advance Social and Economic Well-Being and to Deliver Effective Social Work Services:							
a. Analyze, formulate, and advocate for policies that advance social well-being							
b. Collaborate with colleagues and clients for effective policy action							
EP 2.1.9 Respond to Contexts that Shape Practice:							
a. Continuously discover, appraise, and attend to changing locales, populations, scientific and technological developments, and emerging societal trends to provide relevant services							
b. Provide leadership in promoting sustainable changes in service delivery and practice to improve the quality of social services							
EP 2.1.10 Engage, Assess, Intervene, and Evaluate with Individuals, Families, Groups, Organizations and Communities:							
a. Substantively and affectively prepare for action with individuals, families, groups, organizations, and communities							
b. Use empathy and other interpersonal skills							
c. Develop a mutually agreed-on focus of work and desired outcomes							
d. Collect, organize, and interpret client data							
e. Assess client strengths and limitations							
f. Develop mutually agreed-on intervention goals and objectives							
g. Select appropriate intervention strategies							
h. Initiate actions to achieve organizational goals							
i. Implement prevention interventions that enhance client capacities							
j. Help clients resolve problems							
k. Negotiate, mediate, and advocate for clients							
l. Facilitate transitions and endings							
m. Critically analyze, monitor, and evaluate interventions							

Chapter 16
Sociological Aspects of Later Adulthood

Competencies/Practice Behaviors Exercise 16.1
Keeping the Social Security System Healthy

Focus Competencies or Practice Behaviors:

- EP 2.1.1b Practice personal reflection and self-correction to assure continual professional development
- EP 2.1.6b Use research evidence to inform practice
- EP 2.1.7a Utilize conceptual frameworks to guide the processes of assessment, intervention, and evaluation
- EP 2.1.7b Critique and apply knowledge to understand person and environment
- EP 2.1.8a Analyze, formulate, and advocate for policies that advance social well-being

A. Brief description

You will have small-group discussions aimed at ranking various alternatives for keeping the Social Security system solvent. Findings will then be summarized to the total group and discussed.

B. Objectives

You will:

1. Understand the financial aspects of the Social Security system.
2. Explain to others why the Social Security system in future years may not be able to financially maintain older people.
3. State alternatives for keeping the Social Security system solvent and evaluate the pros and cons of each.

C. Procedure

1. The instructor summarizes information contained in the chapter about: (1) the Social Security system's financial base; (2) there will be more recipients as people live longer; (3) monthly benefit payments are inadequate to totally financially maintain older people, but should they be?; and (4) Social Security taxes have increased dramatically over the years.
2. Form subgroups of five or six persons. Discuss and then rank from 1 to 6 the following alternatives for keeping the Social Security system healthy, with rank number 1 being the most preferred alternative.

Alternatives

a. Continue to raise the maximum tax on Social Security an average of $250 per year. This amount is roughly the current average increase. With this kind of increase, the maximum tax paid in the year 2010 would be $10,000 per employee.

b. Withhold highly expensive medical care from those over age 75. Less expensive medical care would continue to be provided.

c. For those over 85, do not provide medical treatment for life-threatening illnesses, such as cancer, heart attacks, or pneumonia. Treatment for minor ailments, such as colds and arthritis, would continue to be given.

d. Use physician-assisted suicide for those in a nursing home who meet both of the following conditions: (a) have no chance of returning to society, and (b) sincerely express (for at least a two-month period) a wish to die.

e. Sharply reduce the benefits paid out of the Social Security system. (With this approach, many of the current recipients would be deeply impoverished.)

f. Seek to increase the amount of money in the Social Security system by investing available funds in the stock market.

3. A representative from each small group lists the group's rankings on the board. A representative from each group explains the reasons for its rankings. Discuss these rankings.

Competencies/Practice Behaviors Exercise 16.2
Hard Choices About Living Conditions for Older People

Focus Competencies or Practice Behaviors:

- EP 2.1.1b Practice personal reflection and self-correction to assure continual professional development
- EP 2.1.3a Distinguish, appraise, and integrate multiple sources of knowledge, including research-based knowledge and practice wisdom
- EP 2.1.6b Use research evidence to inform practice
- EP 2.1.7a Utilize conceptual frameworks to guide the processes of assessment, intervention, and evaluation
- EP 2.1.7b Critique and apply knowledge to understand person and environment

A. Brief description

You are asked to indicate (anonymously) your personal choices relating to difficult questions about living conditions for older people.

B. Objectives

You will:

1. Have a greater understanding of the complex questions that arise about living conditions for older people.
2. Identify and state your values about living conditions for older people.

C. Procedure

1. The instructor hands out sheets of paper or five-by-seven-inch notecards. Write your answers to the following ten multiple-choice questions on your paper or notecard. <u>Do not</u> sign your name.

QUESTIONS

a. If I were age 70, I would prefer to:
   1) Continue to work to maintain my standard of living
   2) Retire, which would mean a sharp reduction in my standard of living
   3) Uncertain

b. If I were age 75 and had a heart disease that was terminal, I would:
   1) Want a heart transplant to attempt to help me live longer
   2) Prefer the less painful way of saying no to a heart transplant and let nature take its course
   3) Uncertain

c. If I were age 80 and my mental and physical capacities had deteriorated substantially, I would want to:
   1) Be placed in a nursing home
   2) Continue living in my own home, where I would be unlikely to meet my basic needs and therefore might die
   3) Uncertain

d. If I were age 75, I would prefer:
   1) To die fairly suddenly, with my physical and mental capacities still intact
   2) To continue living for 20 more years in a nursing home, with deteriorated mental and physical capacities
   3) Uncertain

e. If I lived in a nursing home from age 80 to age 100, I think it would be ____ to younger taxpayers to have them pay my expenses through the Social Security system.
   1) Fair
   2) Unfair
   3) Uncertain

f. I think it is _____ to sign a living will in which I state that, if I am unconscious (for example, in a coma) and have no chance to return to a life of quality, I do not want heroic medical efforts used to keep me alive.
   1) Desirable
   2) Undesirable
   3) Uncertain

g. If one of my parents dies and the remaining parent becomes fairly disabled physically, I _____ allow that parent to live alone if he or she wanted to even though life-threatening conditions could arise.
   1) Would
   2) Would not
   3) Uncertain

h. I _____ believe that an older person who is terminally ill and in intense pain has an ethical right to commit suicide.
1) Do
2) Do not
3) Uncertain

i. If I were married and had young children, and my only surviving parent became fairly disabled, mentally and physically, I would:
1) Allow the parent to live with me, which would disrupt my family and force family members to provide 24-hour care each day
2) Place the parent in a nursing home
3) Uncertain

j. I think middle-aged adults _____ an obligation to physically take care of their parents, just as parents are obligated to take care of their children.
1) Have
2) Do not have
3) Uncertain

2. Hand in your papers or cards anonymously. The instructor writes on the chalkboard the identifying letters of the questions and the numbers of the possible responses:

	1	2	3
a.			
b.			
c.			
d.			
e.			
f.			
g.			
h.			
i.			
j.			

A volunteer lists the responses.

3. The instructor rereads each question out loud and then leads a discussion about the responses.

Competencies/Practice Behaviors Exercise 16.3
Physician-Assisted Suicide Role-Play

Focus Competencies or Practice Behaviors:

- EP 2.1.1b Practice personal reflection and self-correction to assure continual professional development
- EP 2.1.3a Distinguish, appraise, and integrate multiple sources of knowledge, including research-based knowledge and practice wisdom
- EP 2.1.6b Use research evidence to inform practice
- EP 2.1.7a Utilize conceptual frameworks to guide the processes of assessment, intervention, and evaluation
- EP 2.1.7b Critique and apply knowledge to understand person and environment

A. Brief description

You are asked two questions related to whether you believe physician-assisted suicide should be legalized.

B. Objectives

You will:

1. Identify the arguments on both sides of this issue.
2. Clarify your values on this national issue.

C. Procedure

1. Form subgroups of four or five persons. Each subgroup discusses the following two questions:
   a. If I were 75 years old, had a terminal illness, and were in severe pain, would I consider physician-assisted suicide as being an option for coping with my deteriorating condition? Why or why not?
   b. Should physician-assisted suicide be legalized for older persons who have a terminal illness, are in severe pain, and want to die? Why or why not?
2. A representative from each subgroup shares the diverse views of its members with the class.
3. The instructor ends the exercise by providing a summary of the views that are expressed.

Chapter 16 Competencies/Practice Behaviors Exercises Assessment:

Name: ______________________ **Date:** __________
Supervisor's Name: ______________________

Focus Competencies or Practice Behaviors:

- EP 2.1.1b Practice personal reflection and self-correction to assure continual professional development
- EP 2.1.3a Distinguish, appraise, and integrate multiple sources of knowledge, including research-based knowledge and practice wisdom
- EP 2.1.6b Use research evidence to inform practice
- EP 2.1.7a Utilize conceptual frameworks to guide the processes of assessment, intervention, and evaluation
- EP 2.1.7b Critique and apply knowledge to understand person and environment
- EP 2.1.8a Analyze, formulate, and advocate for policies that advance social well-being

Instructions:

A. Evaluate your work or your partner's work in the Focus Competencies/Practice Behaviors by completing the Competencies/Practice Behaviors Assessment form below

B. What other Competencies/Practice Behaviors did you use to complete these Exercises? Be sure to record them in your assessments

1.	I have attained this competency/practice behavior (in the range of 81 to 100%)
2.	I have largely attained this competency/practice behavior (in the range of 61 to 80%)
3.	I have partially attained this competency/practice behavior (in the range of 41 to 60%)
4.	I have made a little progress in attaining this competency/practice behavior (in the range of 21 to 40%)
5.	I have made almost no progress in attaining this competency/practice behavior (in the range of 0 to 20%)

EPAS 2008 Core Competencies & Core Practice Behaviors	Student Self Assessment						Evaluator Feedback
Student and Evaluator Assessment Scale and Comments	**0**	**1**	**2**	**3**	**4**	**5**	**Agree/Disagree/Comments**
EP 2.1.1 Identify as a Professional Social Worker and Conduct Oneself Accordingly:							
a. Advocate for client access to the services of social work							
b. Practice personal reflection and self-correction to assure continual professional development							
c. Attend to professional roles and boundaries							
d. Demonstrate professional demeanor in behavior, appearance, and communication							
e. Engage in career-long learning							
f. Use supervision and consultation							
EP 2.1.2 Apply Social Work Ethical Principles to Guide Professional Practice:							
a. Recognize and manage personal values in a way that allows professional values to guide practice							